# Management of
# Challenging Behaviors
# in Dementia

# Management of Challenging Behaviors in Dementia

*Ellen K. Mahoney, D.N.S., R.N., C.S.*
*Ladislav Volicer, M.D., Ph.D.*
*Ann C. Hurley, R.N., D.N.S., F.A.A.N., C.N.A.*

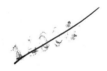

**HEALTH PROFESSIONS PRESS**

Baltimore · London · Winnipeg · Sydney

**Health Professions Press, Inc.**
PO Box 10624
Baltimore, Maryland 21285-0624

www.healthpropress.com

Typeset by PRO-IMAGE Corporation, York, Pennsylvania.
Manufactured in the United States of America by Versa Press, Inc., East Peoria,
Illinois.

**Library of Congress Cataloging-in-Publication Data**
Mahoney, Ellen, 1948–
    Management of challenging behaviors in dementia / Ellen Mahoney, Ladislav
Volicer, Ann C. Hurley.
        p. cm.
    Includes bibliographical references and index.
    ISBN 1-878812-46-7
    1. Dementia—Patients—Care. 2. Dementia—Treatment. I. Volicer, Ladislav. II.
Hurley, Ann, DSc. III. Title

RC521.M344 2000
616.8'3—dc21
                                                                            00-063239
British Cataloguing in Publication Data are available from the British Library.

# Contents

Introduction ..................................................................................................1

Chapter 1    Dementia and Personality .........................................................11

Chapter 2    Functional Impairment .............................................................29

Chapter 3    Mood Disorders.........................................................................47

Chapter 4    Delusions and Hallucinations ...................................................65

Chapter 5    Dependence in Activities of Daily Living ................................79

Chapter 6    Inability to Initiate Meaningful Activities................................93

Chapter 7    Anxiety ...................................................................................109

Chapter 8    Spatial Disorientation..............................................................125

Chapter 9    Resistiveness to Care...............................................................139

Chapter 10   Food Refusal ..........................................................................155

Chapter 11   Insomnia ................................................................................171

Chapter 12   Apathy and Agitation .............................................................187

Chapter 13   Elopement and Interference with Others ...............................205

Glossary......................................................................................................217

Index .........................................................................................................225

# About the Authors

**Ellen K. Mahoney, D.N.S., R.N., C.S.,** is Associate Professor, Boston College School of Nursing, and Senior Research Health Scientist, Geriatric Research Education and Clinical Center (GRECC), Edith Nourse Rogers Veterans Administration Hospital. She is certified as a Gerontological Nurse Specialist by the American Nurses Association Credentialing Center and is a research fellow of the Rehabilitation Nursing Foundation.

Dr. Mahoney did undergraduate work at Georgetown University, received the Master of Science degree from the University of Pennsylvania, and was awarded the Doctorate in Nursing Science by the University of California, San Francisco. She has been formally recognized by Boston College nursing students for excellence in teaching and by clinical staff for excellence in advancing the care of people with dementia.

As a clinical nurse researcher, Dr. Mahoney has received federal and organizational funding for her work on promoting the functional status of older adults with dementia in both community and institutional environments and in evaluating nursing interventions to manage behavioral symptoms in people with dementia. Her publications related to the care of people with dementia focus on instrument development, understanding behavioral symptoms, and symptom management.

**Ladislav Volicer, M.D., Ph.D.,** is Clinical Director of the GRECC and Medical Director of the Dementia Special Care Unit, a 100-bed inpatient unit, at the Edith Nourse Rogers Veterans Administration Hospital. In addition, Dr. Volicer serves as Professor of Pharmacology and Psychiatry and Assistant Professor of Medicine at the Boston University School of Medicine, as a research psychiatrist at McLean Hospital, and as external professor at the 3rd Medical Faculty at Charles University in Prague, Czech Republic.

He received the Doctor of Medicine degree from Charles University School of Medicine and the Doctor of Philosophy degree from the Czechoslovak Academy of Sciences.

Dr. Volicer has edited five books and published more than 170 articles on Alzheimer's disease, neuropharmacology, aging, and bioethics. He has served on numerous grant committees and on the editorial boards of three journals.

**Ann C. Hurley, R.N., D.N.Sc., F.A.A.N., C.N.A.,** is Associate Director for Education and Program Evaluation for the GRECC at the Edith Nourse Rogers Veterans Administration Hospital. She also serves as Adjunct Professor of Nursing at Northeastern University, as a research associate at the Boston University School of Public Health, and as Education Core Leader at the

Boston University Alzheimer Disease Center. Dr. Hurley also is a Colonel in the United States Army Reserve.

She received both her Master of Science and Doctor of Nursing Science from the Boston University School of Nursing. She has received a number of honors, including Distinguished Practitioner of Nursing by the National Academies Practice, Distinguished Nurse Researcher by the Massachusetts Nursing Association, and Fellow of the American Academy of Nursing.

Dr. Hurley has published widely on many topics related to Alzheimer's disease, with a particular focus on instrument development and palliative care management of people with dementia, as well as on the promotion of interdisciplinary grant writing.

# Introduction

People older than age 65 are the largest growing segment of the U.S. population, and aging is the primary risk factor for developing the most prevalent progressive dementia, Alzheimer's disease (Hurley & Wells, 1999a). Between 2.5 and 4 million Americans have Alzheimer's disease, numbers that will continue to increase as the U.S. population ages (AMA Council on Scientific Affairs, 1998). There are 360,000 new Alzheimer's disease cases annually in the United States, and by 2050, 1 in 45 Americans may develop Alzheimer's disease unless a cure is found (Klein & Kowall, 1998). Millions of people will live with dementia even if no new cases occur, and caregivers will continue to need better ways to provide care.

Progressive dementias are terminal illnesses; people with Alzheimer's disease or a related dementia may live for up to 20 years before dying from complications related to dementia. Some medications delay the clinical symptoms of disease progression, but no medication stops the pathological changes or their clinical consequences. Although the pathological processes of dementia cannot yet be halted or reversed, caregivers can manage symptoms and improve the quality of life for people with the disease. Successful management of challenging behaviors in dementia is critical to the well-being of older adults with dementia and their caregivers.

Figure 1 illustrates the contextual framework for understanding challenging behaviors and caregiving strategies that are targeted to symptom management, which forms the foundation of this book (Volicer & Hurley, 1998). Three levels of the framework are distinguished: core, secondary, and peripheral. The dementing process directly causes functional impairment. In combination with the person's underlying personality, the dementing process may cause delusions, hallucinations, and mood disorders. These core conse-

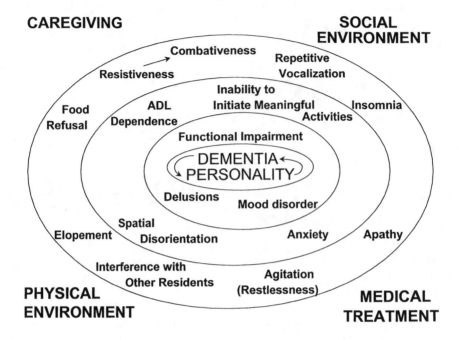

*Figure 1.*

quences lead to secondary symptoms such as spatial disorientation, anxiety, dependence in activities of daily living (ADLs), and inability to initiate meaningful activities. Other behavioral symptoms, such as resistiveness or agitation, are peripheral expressions of the core consequences. Because secondary and peripheral symptoms can be managed more effectively by treating their cause rather than their clinical manifestations, a thorough assessment and evaluation is critical.

Core consequences and secondary symptoms often cause more than one peripheral symptom, and processes at each level of the framework influence the next level comprehensively. For example, delusions may result in spatial disorientation, anxiety, and dependence in ADLs. Depression may result from these symptoms and lead to anxiety and an inability to initiate meaningful activities. Similarly, spatial disorientation may lead to elopement, combativeness, interference with other people, and agitation. The inability to initiate meaningful activities may lead to apathy, repetitive vocalization, agitation, and insomnia.

Conversely, each peripheral symptom can be caused by more than one core consequence or secondary symptom. For example, agitation may be caused by delusions or depression, and attempts at elopement may be the consequence of delusions or spatial disorientation. Therefore, multiple etiologies for specific behavioral symptoms are possible, and therapies are more effective when interventions are directed closer to core consequences. The relationships of the underlying processes to behavioral symptoms may differ from person to person. In fact, they may differ in the same person at different times. Therefore, the effective management of behavioral symptoms requires a careful and comprehensive evaluation of all possible contributing factors. A single challenging behavior does not direct the choice of intervention; interventions are directed by the individual's behavior, the unique characteristics of the individual, and the contexts in which his or her challenging behaviors occur.

Four areas in our model direct symptom management: caregiving, social environment, physical environment, and medical treatment. Caregivers and caregiving strategies are vital to the intervention process, and our philosophical approach is to try nonpharmacological approaches first (Volicer, Mahoney, & Brown, 1998). The philosophy of care that undergirds this book is that giving care to people with a dementing illness is carried out within a hierarchy of safety → comfort → quality of life → dignity. The area of social environment asks caregivers to recognize and accommodate the needs of people with dementia and can range from a one-to-one interaction to a special care program (Volicer & Simard, 1996). The physical environment emphasizes the importance of environmental design, both as an intervention for challenging behaviors in dementia (Zeisel, Hyde, & Shi, 1999) and a "crutch" to help people with dementia compensate for cognitive and functional deficits. Medical treatment ensures that physical problems, whether related or unrelated to dementia, are addressed and treated (Volicer, 1996).

The classification "stage of dementia" is related to how and when associated challenging behaviors appear. Several classification systems have been proposed to describe stages that are observed commonly in the dementing diseases. We find it useful to distinguish four such stages (Figure 2): mild, moderate, severe, and terminal (Volicer & Hurley, 1998). There are several schemes for classifying dementia stages. Our group distinguishes the four stages shown in Figure 2, in which the slope indicates loss of independence over time (Volicer & Hurley, 1998). As the disease progresses, the person first loses the ability to perform independently instrumental ADLs (IADLs) and gradually becomes completely dependent in all aspects of ADLs (Hurley, Volicer, & Mahoney, 1996). Dementia can affect different areas of the brain. Therefore, the course and symptoms are highly variable, and the person may live from 2 to 20 years after diagnosis (Hurley & Wells, 1999b). The use of four stages—from mild to terminal—recognizes that Alzheimer's disease is both a chronic and life-limiting disorder. All people are unique and people with Alzheimer's disease, even identical twins, will have different clinical symptoms at different times. In fact, people may experience symptoms that are characteristic of several stages simultaneously.

Instead of attempting to label an individual by a specific stage number,

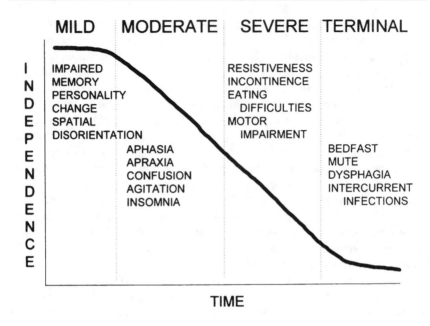

*Figure 2.*

which is artificial at best, the slope indicates progression through four general stages. Caregiver involvement may be drawn as an inverse of the slope because as the person with dementia loses independence and develops specific symptoms, caregivers must intervene more to compensate for those losses and for the development of behavioral symptoms.

Although our focus is nonpharmacological interventions, we also want to direct attention to pharmacotherapies. Appropriate medications, including their intended effects and their side effects, are examined in the chapters that follow. Medication selection that is based on the balance between therapeutic effects and side-effect profiles that would be the least problematic for the person with dementia is described. (Medications are prescribed solely for the *comfort* of the person with dementia and for no other reason.) The management of side effects, dosage adjustments, and "golden rules" to follow when pharmacotherapy is indicated also are discussed. Particular emphasis is placed on the avoidance of polypharmacy and on the need to start with a low dose that is increased slowly.

Caring for the person with dementia is an art and a science. The art requires respectful and educated caregivers who provide person-centered care. The science requires evidence-based care that is applied by following objective standards, treatment guidelines, and outcome criteria. The chapters present caregiving strategies that work across the continuum of care. Case studies focus on the perspective of the person with dementia to illustrate specific points related to nursing, medical and behavioral management, the social and physical environments, and caregiving strategies.

The book consists of 13 chapters, one for each component of our model (Figure 1), and a glossary of terms used in the text. Every chapter describes a case study illustrating the chapter's topic. All case studies are fictitious and use names that correspond by letter of the alphabet with the chapter number. The authors recognize that an autopsy examination may find evidence for more than one cause of dementia, that the relative contribution of these causes to the clinical syndrome is unclear, and that some clinical differences are observed among the progressive dementing disorders. However, in this book, we generally use the diagnosis of Alzheimer's disease because it is the most prevalent dementia, or we refer to "the person with dementia" because behavioral symptoms are similar in many progressive dementias. We point out when a specific behavioral problem occurs more commonly or earlier in the disease process in another dementing disorder.

Chapter 1 employs the case study of Mrs. Alva, who presents with changes in personality, to guide the reader through an overview of the most common of the acquired dementing disorders from initial differential diagnosis to available treatment. Dementia is distinguished from delirium. The components of a complete diagnostic dementia workup are described, and strategies for differentiation of Alzheimer's disease, vascular disease, dementia with Lewy bodies, and frontotemporal dementia are presented. Genetic and environmental factors that may cause Alzheimer's disease and risk factors for developing Alzheimer's disease are identified. The roles of hormone replacement therapy, free radical scavengers, and cholinesterase inhibitors as therapeutics for Alzheimer's disease are discussed.

Chapters 2–4 present the model's three primary consequences of dementia. Chapter 2 uses the case study of Mrs. Browne to describe functional impairment, which is determined by two interactive components of this core consequence, cognitive and physical impairment. The assessment of cognitive function is presented by describing the standard tests used and including the perspective of a person with mild dementia who knows that she cannot answer the questions that are posed to her. Short-term memory and executive function losses are described. Examples are given to describe the "A" deficits in dementia—aphasia, apraxia, and agnosia. Intervention strategies for cognitive impairment for people in mild to severe stages are presented. Physical impairment and the relationships among dementia, immobility, and comorbidity are discussed. Intervention strategies to delay or minimize physical impairment in mild to moderate, moderate to severe, and terminal stages of dementing illness are presented. Principles of communication strategies are outlined.

Chapter 3 is an examination of mood disorders. Mrs. Clarke's depressive symptoms are used to illustrate the epidemiology and types of mood disorders. Depressive disorders including major depressive disorder, dysthymic disorder, adjustment disorder with depressed mood, and depressive disorders not otherwise specified are discussed, as is bipolar disorder. Treatment options for mood disorders such as the use of antidepressants, psychotherapy, electroconvulsive therapy, and mood stabilizers are explained. The relationships between mood disorders and dementia are explored, and specific combinations of these comorbidities are presented. The consequences of depression in advanced dementia are described. Three tables that list diagnostic criteria, antidepressant medications, and mood stabilizers are included.

The case study in Chapter 4 presents the conditions that cause delusions and hallucinations, their epidemiology and etiology, and the relationship of delusions and hallucinations to other behavioral symptoms of dementia. An outline of interventions that use environmental and communication strategies to prevent or decrease delusions and hallucinations by nonpharmacological approaches is provided. Because delusions and hallucinations may require pharmacological intervention, drug therapy is discussed and a table of selected medications used in the treatment of delusions and hallucinations is presented.

Four secondary symptoms are discussed in Chapters 5–8. Chapter 5 follows Mrs. Ewing from the assessment of her capacity to perform IADLs and physical ADLs to the selection of interventions that are aimed at decreasing her dependence. Core consequences, contextual factors, and risk factors for functional decline are examined in terms of the etiology for problems in performing ADLs. Interventions to promote function in the areas of IADLs and bathing, dressing, toileting/continence, and eating are presented. Examples of IADL adaptations are provided, and strategies to promote functional performance are listed.

"Inability to Initiate Meaningful Activities," Chapter 6, uses the case study of Mr. Franklin to illustrate the definition, characteristics, and risk factors for this secondary symptom. Guidelines for the choice of activities, selected interventions depending on the stage of dementia, and documentation of treatment effectiveness are presented. Interventions for mild to moderate dementia include cognitive activity, functional household activities, diversional activities, reminiscence, Video Respite®, and exercise. Interventions for moderate to severe dementia include simulated presence therapy, music, Bright Eyes, reminiscence, pets, Merry Walker, and Snoezelen.

Chapter 7 cites instances from the case study of Mrs. Gomez to define anxiety and to illustrate the assessment of anxiety, anxiety in older adults, and anxiety coupled with dementia. An explanatory model of anxiety illustrates the effects of three etiologies/risk factors of emotional response, medical causes, and psychiatric symptoms on outcomes. Primary anxiety disorders, anxiety as a symptom of illness, and anxiety as a stress response are differentiated. Medical conditions and medications that can produce symptoms of anxiety, clinical indicators of anxiety, and interventions to promote minimal levels of stress are listed. Three types of interventions to achieve therapeutic goals are presented. Environment-focused interventions to prevent anxiety include encouraging minimal levels of stress, enhancing feelings of trust and safety, and promoting control. Behavioral interventions include music therapy, reminiscence, and Snoezelen. Pharmacological treatment is discussed, and guidelines for the initiation of anxiolytic medications and selected drugs to treat anxiety are included.

The chapter on spatial disorientation "walks the walk" of a disoriented man with dementia, Mr. Henley, using the analogy of the "Wizard of Alz," and provides the rationale for interventions to manage spatial disorientation. Pathophysiological causes and bases for interventions are described. A model to help readers understand spatial disorientation places this secondary symptom in the center and illustrates relationships among the antecedents and effects related to this behavioral symptom. Specific management suggestions for spatial disorientation for mild, moderate, and severe dementia are listed.

Five peripheral symptoms are discussed in Chapters 9–13. Chapter 9, "Resistiveness to Care," defines and identifies the properties of resistive behaviors using the case study of Mr. Ingram. A behavioral model of resistiveness to care depicts relationships among antecedents, behaviors, and consequences. The assessment of patients at risk for resistiveness is discussed in terms of care recipient and caregiver variables and context of care. Use of behavioral and pharmacological interventions to prevent and manage symptoms are discussed. Resistiveness to care during bathing is explained in detail, and recommended environmental characteristics for bathing areas and procedures for using a gentle towel bath are listed.

Chapter 10 follows Mrs. Jeng as general guidelines to promote eating and prevent food refusal are presented. Specific eating problems that are caused by dementia are discussed, and the three components of establishing a nourishment plan—planning food/nutrition, establishing eating areas, and shaping the eating process—are described. Strategies for managing food refusal through the four progressive stages of mild, moderate, severe, and terminal dementia and characteristics of food to promote safe eating are listed. Two tables, "Managing Food Refusal" and "Preventing/Breaking Cycle of Behaviors Used to Refuse Food," provide suggested approaches to intervene when food is refused. Evidence is presented to correct widely held misconceptions about feeding tubes, which are sometimes used to manage the consequences of food refusal in the terminal stage of dementia.

Using the case study of Mr. Kupfer, Chapter 11 lists the stages of sleep with predominant electroencephalogram waves and eye movements and describes the regulation of sleep. Three major conditions affecting sleep—sleep-related respiratory disorders, sleep-related motor disorders, and medical conditions that are common in older adults—are discussed. A model illustrates the interaction of age, dementia, and environmental factors in the development of insomnia. The effects of dementia on sleep in terms of stages of sleep and sleep-related disorders and the effects of depression and anxiety on sleep are discussed. The treatment of insomnia through lifestyle changes, behavioral methods of stimulus control instructions and sleep restriction therapy, chronobiological strategies, and pharmacological treatment are presented. Interventions, including stimulus control strategies for people with dementia, are examined.

Chapter 12, "Agitation and Apathy," differentiates apathy from depression and discusses engagement using examples from the case study of Mrs. Luke. A model of psychological well-being that is specific to people with dementia that includes agitation and apathy as central concepts illustrates how the worsening of dementia over time restricts the range of and capacity to express emotions. Physical causes of agitation and depression are discussed, and the rationale for therapeutics is presented. Medications, caregiving strategies, simulated presence therapy, and sundown syndrome are examined. Three tables list approaches to assess the possible causes of agitation, general guidelines to prevent or minimize the agitated behaviors of the person with dementia, and general guidelines to manage the agitated behaviors of the person with dementia.

Finally, Chapter 13 follows Mrs. Minkiezich to describe wandering and both person- and environment-focused interventions to prevent elopement. A model illustrates how underlying causes plus the presence of precipitants can change harmless wandering behaviors into the serious problem of elopement. The advantages of walking and pacing are described, and interventions to provide safe wandering are presented.

# REFERENCES

AMA Council on Scientific Affairs, Reference Committee D. (1998). Alzheimer's disease. *Journal of the American Medical Association, 91*(5), 298–306.

Hurley, A.C., & Wells, N. (1999a). Past, present, and future directions for Alzheimer research. *Alzheimer Disease and Associated Disorders, 13*, S6–S10.

Hurley, A.C., & Wells, N. (1999b). Nursing research and solving problems of Alzheimer disease. *Alzheimer Disease and Associated Disorders, 13*, S73–S77.

Hurley, A.C., Volicer, L., & Mahoney, E. (1996, March). Progression of Alzheimer's disease and symptom management. *Federal Practitioner,* S16–S22.

Klein, A., & Kowall, N. (1998). Alzheimer's disease and other progressive dementias. In L. Volicer & A.C. Hurley (Eds.), *Hospice care for patients with advanced progressive dementia* (pp. 3–28). New York: Springer.

Volicer, L. (1996). Clinical issues in advanced dementia. In S.B. Hoffman & M. Kaplan (Eds.), *Special care programs for people with dementia* (pp. 61–77). Baltimore: Health Professions Press.

Volicer, L., & Hurley, A. (Eds.). (1998). *Hospice care for patients with advanced progressive dementia.* New York: Springer.

Volicer, L., Mahoney, E., & Brown, E.J. (1998). Nonpharmacological approaches to the management of the behavioral consequences of advanced dementia. In M. Kaplan & S.B. Hoffman (Eds.), *Behaviors in dementia: Best practices for successful management.* (pp. 155–176). Baltimore: Health Professions Press.

Volicer, L., & Simard, J. (1996). Establishing a dementia special-care unit. *Nursing Home Economics, 3*(1), 12–19.

Zeisel, J., Hyde, J., & Shi, L. (1999). Environmental design as a treatment for Alzheimer's disease. In L. Volicer & L. Bloom-Charett (Eds.), *Enhancing quality of life in advanced dementia* (pp. 206–222). Philadelphia: Taylor & Francis.

# 1

# Dementia and Personality

Dementia is an acquired syndrome that causes the progressive loss of intellectual abilities, such as memory, language (*aphasia*), and the person's ability to use tools (*apraxia*), to recognize objects (*agnosia*), and to plan and think in abstract terms (loss of *executive function*). Dementia is present if at least memory and one additional intellectual ability are impaired and if the impairment is severe enough to interfere with social or occupational functioning (American Psychiatric Association, 1994). If a person exhibits symptoms of dementia, then he or she should be evaluated to determine its causes.

## DEMENTIA AND DELIRIUM

An impairment of cognitive function may be caused not only by the development of dementia but also by delirium. It is important to eliminate delirium as a cause of cognitive impairment because cognitive impairment caused by delirium may be reversible. Delirium is characterized by an acute onset of mental status change (fluctuating course; decreased ability to focus, sustain, and shift attention; and either disorganized thinking or an altered level of consciousness) that resolves if the precipitating causes are removed. The diagnosis of delirium, however, is not easy because some of these diagnostic criteria

11

are not unique to delirium (Macdonald & Treloar, 1996). Acute onset of mental status change also may be caused by vascular dementia. A fluctuating course of cognitive impairment is an important clinical diagnostic feature of dementia with Lewy bodies (McKeith et al., 1996). The concept of delirium as a transient cognitive impairment is challenged by a study indicating that cognitive impairment resolves within 3 months in only 20% of people with a diagnosis of delirium (Levkoff et al., 1992).

The prevalence of disorganized thinking expressed by delusions and hallucinations is similar in people with reversible and irreversible cognitive dysfunction. Specific symptoms of reversible dysfunction include plucking at bedclothes; poor attention; incoherent speech; abnormal associations; and slow, vague thoughts (Treloar & Macdonald, 1997b). The criteria for delirium in the *Diagnostic and Statistical Manual of Mental Disorders, Fourth Edition, Revised* (American Psychiatric Association, 1994) do not predict improvement in cognitive function in all cases, and the Reversible Cognitive Dysfunction Scale, which accurately predicts improvement, has been devised (Treloar & Macdonald, 1997a).

Delirium may be precipitated by many medical conditions (e.g., infections, dehydration, metabolic disorder) and adverse effects of medications (e.g., drugs that have an anticholinergic effect, such as diphenhydramine, thioridazine, and benztropine; cardiac medications, such as digoxin and antihypertensive agents; drugs used to treat peptic ulcers, such as cimetidine). Regardless of the cause, the development of delirium may indicate decreased reserve capacity of the brain and may signal an increased risk for dementia (Reifler, 1997). Dementia is a risk factor for delirium, and delirium may contribute to excess disability in individuals with dementia. Therefore, the possibility that delirium is responsible for the onset of new behavioral symptoms always should be considered.

## PERSONALITY CHANGES

The first symptom of dementia usually is short-term memory impairment. In some individuals, however, the first symptom of dementia that is recognized by family members may be impairment of driving ability, language difficulties, or inability to maintain family finances. Early stages of dementia often are not recognized if the individual is retired because he or she is not required to use the higher intellectual capacity that is essential in a work setting. Similarly, people who live in a sheltered environment, such as assisted living or a nursing facility, may have a delayed diagnosis of dementia because their impairments are not obvious in the absence of a challenging environment or of the need to use higher-order intellectual capacity. In some cases the first symptom of dementia is a change in personality.

Mrs. Alba is a 59-year-old waitress who has become less outgoing and less interested in her needlework and cooking. Instead of her usual easygoing personality, she has begun to worry about the future, and instead of her typical easygoing approach to the world, she has become irritable. She denies having any problems and does not want to seek help. Her family is worried and has tried to persuade her to see a physician. After an intensive effort by all family members, Mrs. Alba agrees to see her primary care physician, but insists that she go by herself.

Personality changes occur in all progressive dementias, but they are characterized best in individuals with Alzheimer's disease, which is the most common cause of dementia (Chatterjee, Strauss, Smyth, & Whitehouse, 1992). People with Alzheimer's disease develop neurotic, less extroverted, and less conscientious behaviors. Neurotic behaviors in people with Alzheimer's disease include worrying about things that previously would not have bothered the person; being apprehensive; experiencing anger, irritability, and hatred; feeling hopeless, guilty, and sad; feeling shame and embarrassment; and being dependent on others. Decreased extroversion leads to a diminished tendency to seek emotional ties, less energetic and active behavior, and a decreased tendency to seek stimulation and experience positive emotions. Decreased conscientiousness is expressed by the tendency to be less organized, diligent, and reliable.

In general, people with early-stage Alzheimer's disease still retain many abilities, but they have a decreased appreciation of art and beauty. They are less intellectually curious and open-minded, and their imagination becomes more vivid. These personality changes occur in most individuals and are not dependent on the personality the person had before developing dementia. Despite these changes, however, people with dementia tend to maintain their unique pattern of premorbid personality traits (Kolanowski & Whall, 1996). The personality changes induced by dementia may be quite subtle and difficult to detect during an examination. If the primary provider does not have previous knowledge of the person and does not take into consideration family reports of personality changes, then the initial stages of dementia often are missed.

Personality changes in other types of dementia depend on the areas of the brain that are affected by the disease. Individuals with frontotemporal dementia exhibit loss of social or personal awareness, disinhibited behavior, or disengagement with apathy (Kertesz, Davidson, & Fox, 1997). Similar personality changes occur if an individual experiences a stroke that affects the frontal lobes of the brain. Wandering may be related to impairment of parietal lobe function, and left-sided metabolic reduction in brain function is associated with anxiety-tension, hostility, and depression (Kolanowski & Whall, 1996).

The primary care physician does not find any medical problems in Mrs. Alba during standard physical examination and interpretation of laboratory results. Thinking that the complaints are the result of stress, the care provider recommends to Mrs. Alba that she work fewer hours. Mrs. Alba starts working part-time, but her personality problems do not ameliorate. Six months later, Mrs. Alba experiences difficulty remembering the items on the menu, makes mistakes in customers' orders, and cannot total their bills. The rest of her family insists that Mrs. Alba see the doctor again and that her daughter Allison go with her. After Allison explains the problems Mrs. Alba has been experiencing, the physician refers Mrs. Alba to a neurologist.

A neurological examination detects a slight memory deficit and impairment in spatial orientation but does not find any evidence of abnormal reflexes or nerve functions that indicate damage to a specific part of the brain. Mrs. Alba's diagnostic workup includes additional laboratory tests, but the results are within normal limits. Brain imaging by magnetic resonance imaging (MRI), however, shows brain atrophy, and an electroencephalogram shows diffuse slowing of brain function. The neurologist also requests a detailed examination of cognitive functioning (a standard battery of tests to make a neuropsychological evaluation) that shows concrete interpretation of proverbs (e.g., "the grass is always greener on the other side of the fence" is explained literally), and deficits in word generation and visuospatial memory.

## DIAGNOSTIC WORKUP IN DEMENTIA

The two purposes of the diagnostic workup are the exclusion of potentially reversible causes of dementia and the initiation of therapy as early as possible. A variety of conditions may cause the syndrome of dementia. When these conditions are detected early enough, some of them may be reversible (Table 1.1). Unfortunately, the number of people whose symptoms of dementia are successfully treated and reversed is rather small. A review of 870 patients seen at a memory disorder clinic indicated that 11% had a cause of dementia for which some therapy was available, but in most patients the dementia was not reversed despite the appropriate treatment (Alzheimer's Disease and Related Dementia Guideline Panel, 1996).

A diagnostic workup also may show that a person is not demented. The Alzheimer's Disease and Related Dementia Guideline Panel (1996) reported that another 15% of patients were found not to have dementia, despite their complaints about memory problems. It is recognized that memory becomes somewhat impaired during normal aging, although this impairment does not interfere with ADLs. Memory impairment caused by normal aging that does not progress is called benign senile forgetfulness (Carlesimo et al., 1998). It is

**Table 1.1.    Some causes of potentially reversible dementias**

Tumors: both in brain and peripheral tissues
Metabolic disorders: thyroid disease, electrolyte imbalance, renal or hepatic failure
Head trauma
Poisoning: heavy metals, alcoholism, solvents, and insecticides
Brain infections
Autoimmune disorders: brain vasculitis, lupus erythematosus, multiple sclerosis
Adverse effects of drugs
Nutritional disorders: deficiency of vitamins $B_{12}$, $B_6$, $B_1$, and folate
Psychiatric disorders
Normal-pressure hydrocephalus
Acquired immunodeficiency syndrome encephalopathy

sometimes difficult to distinguish the early stages of Alzheimer's disease from benign senile forgetfulness. The main difference is that benign senile forgetfulness does not become steadily worse, whereas the hallmark of Alzheimer's disease is the progression of cognitive impairment.

Many individuals with Alzheimer's disease are unaware of their deficits or underestimate the extent of their impairment (*anosognosia*). The degree of unawareness varies with the nature of the impairment. These individuals are for the most part unaware of their memory problems and self-care deficits, whereas they are likely to recognize symptoms if they are anxious, irritable, or depressed (Vasterling, Seltzer, Foss, & Vanderbrook, 1995). In general, people with Alzheimer's disease are brought to a physician for an examination by their relatives who recognize that there is a problem, although the person may deny any memory deficit. Typically, individuals with benign senile forgetfulness seek assessment themselves.

The largest number of patients seen at a memory clinic typically have an irreversible dementia, and the most common irreversible dementia is Alzheimer's disease. The study by the Alzheimer's Disease and Related Dementia Guideline Panel (1996) found that Alzheimer's disease accounted for 66% of all dementia cases. Irreversible dementias have many causes (Table 1.2). It is sometimes difficult to distinguish different progressive dementias by clinical examination for two reasons:

1.  Dementia may be caused by more than one mechanism in the same individual. It is not uncommon that an autopsy examination finds evidence for more than one cause of dementia, and the relative contribution of these causes to the clinical syndrome is unclear. The most common combination is that of Alzheimer's disease and vascular dementia, and the second most common is Alzheimer's disease and dementia with Lewy bodies (Figure 1.1).

2.  The symptoms of all progressive dementias are similar, especially in the later stages of the disease. People may differ in the onset and severity of a

particular symptom; for example, hallucinations may occur early in dementia with Lewy bodies and only later in Alzheimer's disease. In addition, there is no uniform progression of symptoms in any of the dementing illnesses; that is, the symptoms do not appear at a consistent time and in the same order.

## DIAGNOSIS OF ALZHEIMER'S DISEASE

The diagnostic criteria for Alzheimer's disease include multiple cognitive deficits manifested by both memory impairment and at least one other cognitive disturbance (e.g., aphasia, apraxia, agnosia, disturbance of executive function). The cognitive deficits must be severe enough to cause significant impairment in social or occupational functioning and must represent a significant decline from a previous level of functioning. The course of the dementing disorder is characterized by gradual onset and continuing cognitive decline, and the cognitive impairment cannot result from other brain disease, systemic disturbances that can cause dementia (Table 1.1), or drug-induced effects. The possibility that the deficit is caused by other conditions, such as delirium or depression, also must be excluded (see Chapter 3).

Clinical diagnosis of progressive dementias is tentative and needs to be supported by neuropathological examination of the brain. Thus the most definite clinical diagnosis of Alzheimer's disease is "probable Alzheimer's disease," which is made when there are no other possible etiological factors. The neuropathological criteria for Alzheimer's disease include the presence of senile, or neuritic, plaques and neurofibrillary tangles. The plaques and tangles each contain a specific protein that may play a role in the pathogenesis of Alzheimer's disease. β-Amyloid protein is present in the plaques, and the tau protein is found in the tangles. Measurement of these proteins in the cere-

**Table 1.2.    Some causes of irreversible dementias**

Neurogenerative diseases: Alzheimer's disease
Dementia with Lewy bodies
Frontotemporal dementia
Pick's disease
Huntington's disease
Parkinson's disease
Progressive supranuclear palsy
Vascular dementias: multi-infarct dementia
Binswanger's disease
Occlusive cerebrovascular disease
Cerebral embolism
Anoxia secondary to cardiac arrest or carbon monoxide poisoning
Infections: Creutzfeld-Jacob disease
Postencephalitic dementia

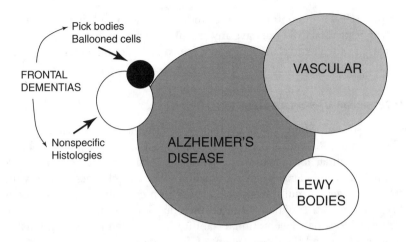

*Figure 1.1. Primary causes of progressive dementia; size of circles indicates the relataive proportion of each as a cause. (From Knopman, D., Schneider, L., Davis, K., Talwalker, S., Smith, F., Hoover, T., & Gracon, S. [1996]. Long-term tacrine [Cognex] treatment: Effects on nursing home placement and mortality. Neurology, 47, 166–177; reprinted by permission.)*

brospinal fluid (CSF) can help to rule out or confirm the diagnosis of Alzheimer's disease in some patients, but it does not give clear-cut results in others (Kanai et al., 1998). Therefore, CSF examination is not recommended as a standard diagnostic test.

Another test that may support the clinical diagnosis of Alzheimer's disease is determination of the apolipoprotein E phenotype. Among individuals who develop Alzheimer's disease, those who have the apolipoprotein E4 phenotype are more likely to develop Alzheimer's disease earlier than individuals who have the apolipoprotein E3 or E2 phenotypes. Not all individuals with apolipoprotein E4 develop dementia however, and most people with dementia have apolipoprotein E3 because this is the most common form of the allele in the general population. Therefore, determination of the apolipoprotein E phenotype provides only limited information, and the determination is not recommended for healthy individuals (American College of Medical Genetics, 1995).

Neuritic plaques and neurofibrillary tangles are present in small quantities even in the brains of elderly individuals who did not have dementia before they died. This finding indicates that formation of plaques and tangles may be a part of the normal aging process and that not everybody who develops plaques and tangles develops dementia. Sister Mary, a nun who was cognitively intact 8 months before her death at age 101, had enough plaques and tangles in her brain on autopsy to warrant a pathological diagnosis of Alzheimer's disease

(Snowdon, 1997). In contrast to other individuals who had dementia before they died, Sister Mary did not have any vascular changes in her brain. Her case demonstrates the close relationship between Alzheimer's disease and vascular dementia.

## DIAGNOSIS OF VASCULAR DEMENTIA

There are several different sets of diagnostic criteria for vascular dementia (Verhey, Lodder, Rozendaal, & Jolles, 1996). Most criteria require an abrupt onset of dementia, focal neurological findings (abnormal reflexes or nerve functions), and low-density areas (indicating vascular changes in the white matter), presence of multiple strokes, or both on computerized tomography (CT) scans or MRI. Other criteria include fluctuation of impairment, unchanged personality, emotional lability, and a temporal relationship between a stroke and the development of dementia.

It must be recognized, however, that vascular changes often are present together with Alzheimer-type changes during brain autopsy. Results of the nun study (Snowdon et al., 1997) indicate that dementia is more severe if both Alzheimer-type and vascular changes are present. The results also show that some individuals who have no vascular changes do not develop dementia despite extensive Alzheimer's-type changes found at autopsy. Thus, it is difficult to exclude the possibility that a person has Alzheimer's disease even when several criteria for vascular dementia are met.

## DIAGNOSIS OF DEMENTIA WITH LEWY BODIES

Dementia with Lewy bodies (also called diffuse Lewy body disease) is characterized by a fluctuating course of cognitive impairment that includes episodic confusion and lucid intervals similar to delirium (McKeith et al., 1994). In addition, there must be at least one of the following: 1) visual or auditory hallucinations, or both, resulting in paranoid delusions; 2) mild extrapyramidal symptoms (e.g., muscle rigidity, slow movements) or adverse extrapyramidal response to standard doses of neuroleptics; or 3) repeated unexplained falls. The clinical features of dementia with Lewy bodies persist over a long period of time, in contrast to delirium, which usually is shorter. Furthermore, dementia with Lewy bodies progresses to severe dementia. As with Alzheimer's disease, other causes of progressive cognitive decline must be excluded.

Dementia with Lewy bodies is characterized during autopsy by the presence of round structures, called Lewy bodies, that are found inside the nerve cells in the brain cortex. These Lewy bodies also are present in Parkinson's disease, but they are limited to subcortical areas of the brain.

## DIAGNOSIS OF FRONTOTEMPORAL DEMENTIA

Frontotemporal dementia, which accounts for up to 10% of all cases of progressive degenerative dementia, has no uniform terminology (Mendez et al., 1996). Some investigators label all frontotemporal dementias "Pick's disease," whereas others consider Pick's disease to be a pathological subtype of frontotemporal dementia, which is characterized by the specific neuropathological findings of Pick's bodies inside nerve cells and ballooned nerve cells. The diagnosis of frontotemporal dementia is based on personality changes and the presence of frontal brain area atrophy in neuroimaging studies (CT or MRI). The personality changes in frontotemporal dementia are similar to changes that are induced by damage to the frontal lobes by other causes (e.g., injury, stroke) and include behavioral disinhibition, loss of social or personal awareness, and disengagement with apathy. People with frontotemporal dementia differ from people with Alzheimer's disease because they retain some abilities (e.g., elementary drawing and calculations) into the later stages of dementia.

Atrophy of the brain's frontal and temporal lobes and proliferation of nonneuronal glial cells in these areas characterize pathological findings in frontotemporal dementia. There are no biochemical tests to help a clinician make the diagnosis of dementia with Lewy bodies or frontotemporal dementia.

On the basis of the clinical evaluation, laboratory, and other studies, Mrs. Alba was diagnosed with probable Alzheimer's disease. Medication therapy was initiated (see "Acetylcholinesterase Inhibitors" later in this chapter).

# CAUSES OF ALZHEIMER'S DISEASE

Alzheimer's disease is very complex and, at this time, knowledge of its causes is limited.

## GENETIC FACTORS

Genetic research indicates that clinical and pathological features of Alzheimer's disease have multiple causes because several genes are involved. Mutations of three genes (on chromosomes 1, 14, and 21) cause Alzheimer's disease in all individuals who have these mutations, and it occurs in half of their children. These mutations involve the formation or metabolism of β-amyloid protein. This protein is present in senile plaques and is toxic to nerve cells. According to one hypothesis, the abnormal formation or metabolism of this protein is the cause of Alzheimer's disease. In cases with these mutations, Alzheimer's disease usually starts quite early, when people are in their 40s and

50s. Only approximately 5% of people with Alzheimer's disease, however, have these mutations (Tilley, Morgan, & Kalsheker, 1998). In the majority of individuals, Alzheimer's disease is related to several genetic and environmental factors. Some of these factors stimulate the development of Alzheimer's disease, whereas other factors may be protective against developing it.

One of the predisposing genetic factors is polymorphism of the gene for apolipoprotein E (located on chromosome 19), mentioned previously. This gene may be responsible for up to 50% of the total genetic influences regarding the predisposition to the development of Alzheimer's disease (Corder et al., 1993). Another genetic factor is related to the major histocompatibility complex, located on chromosome 6, which is involved in inflammation. One form of this complex increases the risk of Alzheimer's disease, whereas another form increases the risk of rheumatoid arthritis. This dichotomy may explain why Alzheimer's disease is less common in people with rheumatoid arthritis than in the general population (Curran et al., 1997). Epidemiological data indicate that people who are taking anti-inflammatory drugs to treat rheumatoid arthritis are less likely to develop Alzheimer's disease. On the basis of these data, it was proposed that anti-inflammatory drugs might be useful in the prevention and treatment of Alzheimer's disease (McGeer, Schulzer, & McGeer, 1996). The alternative explanation is that people with rheumatoid arthritis are less likely to develop Alzheimer's disease because of the chromosome 6 polymorphism than are people without arthritis, regardless of the medication they take. Another genetic factor may be the gene for $\alpha_2$-macroglobulin, located on chromosome 12 (Liao et al., 1998), and other genetic factors may be located on chromosomes 4 and 20 (Pericak-Vance et al., 1997). This is an extremely active area of research that will be helped by the results of the Human Genome Project.

## ENVIRONMENTAL FACTORS

Environmental factors that increase the risk of Alzheimer's disease include head trauma, low education level, estrogen deficiency, early life experiences, and possibly some environmental toxins.

### Head Trauma

A history of head trauma is more common in people with Alzheimer's disease than in controls without dementia, and the effect of brain trauma is more pronounced in individuals carrying the apolipoprotein E4 allele (Mayeux et al., 1995). In some individuals, head trauma occurred long before any clinical symptoms of dementia, and the relationship of trauma to the development of dementia is not clear. However, brain trauma was reported to increase the concentration of $\beta$-amyloid protein in the CSF (Raby et al., 1998). Thus, it is possible that brain trauma leads to the chronic loss of brain cells mediated by the toxic effect of β-amyloid protein.

## Low Level of Education

A low level of education is another risk factor for Alzheimer's disease, and may represent a combination of genetic and environmental influences. Several studies reported that Alzheimer's disease is more common in individuals with less education than in individuals with more education (Mortimer & Graves, 1993). Possible explanations of this difference are earlier detection of dementia in individuals with lower levels of education, who are less able to compensate for a cognitive deficit, or lower brain reserve in individuals having less education, resulting from fewer connections between brain nerve cells. The reserve theory is supported by a finding that Alzheimer's disease progresses faster in individuals with small head circumference than in individuals with larger heads (Graves et al., 1996). This finding indicates that the reserve brain capacity, which may be related to brain size, determines the course of Alzheimer's disease.

## Estrogen Deficiency

Epidemiological evidence indicates that estrogen deficiency increases and hormone replacement therapy in postmenopausal women decreases the risk for Alzheimer's disease (Paganini-Hill & Henderson, 1996). Women on hormone replacement therapy had few pathological changes in the brain white matter detected by MRI. Estrogen could be working as a growth factor, improving connections between nerve cells by interacting with apolipoprotein E or by modifying the metabolism of β-amyloid protein. In cell culture experiments estrogen prevented the toxic effect of β-amyloid protein on nerve cells.

## Early Life Experiences

Evidence is increasing that the development of dementia is influenced by factors that occur in early life. For instance, although people with Alzheimer's disease in general have a higher number of psychosocial stress factors than are found in the general population, one of the factors that is significantly more common in these individuals is that they have lost a parent before age 16. In addition, a study demonstrated that the development of Alzheimer's disease in elderly nuns can be predicted on the basis of the linguistic abilities that were expressed when the nuns were in their 20s (Snowdon et al., 1996).

## Environmental Toxins

The role of environmental toxins is not clear. A correlation has been drawn between the prevalence of Alzheimer's disease and aluminum content in drinking water (Martyn, Coggon, Inksip, Lacey, & Young, 1997), but people exposed to aluminum because they take antacids or work in bauxite mines do not have a higher incidence of the disease. One toxic environmental factor that seems to protect against Alzheimer's disease is smoking. The prevalence of Alzheimer's disease is lower in smokers than in nonsmokers (Lee, 1994). This effect is probably mediated by exposure to nicotine because nicotinic receptors are decreased in individuals with Alzheimer's disease, and exposure to nicotine may make nicotinic receptors more resistant. Smoking has too many adverse health effects, however, to be considered an advisable preventive strategy.

## PREVENTION AND TREATMENT OF ALZHEIMER'S DISEASE

No treatments reverse or stop the advancement of any progressive dementia. Many individual investigators and pharmaceutical companies, however, are trying to find drugs that reverse or slow the clinical symptoms in these conditions. Most efforts are targeted at developing a treatment for Alzheimer's disease, the most common progressive dementia. Some of the treatments used for Alzheimer's disease, however, also may be useful in other progressive dementias. The efforts to develop treatments are guided by contemporary knowledge of the changes in brain chemistry that are induced by the disease and by epidemiological information regarding the relationship between dementia and other conditions.

### HORMONE REPLACEMENT THERAPY

Alzheimer's disease is less common among women who were taking hormone replacement therapy (Yaffe, Sawaya, Lieberburg, & Grady, 1998). A well-controlled double-blind study found, however, that estrogen replacement therapy for 1 year did not slow the progression of the disease nor did it improve cognitive or functional status of women with mild to moderate Alzheimer's disease (Mulnard et al., 2000). Hormone replacement therapy is recommended for all women who have had a hysterectomy and bilateral oophorectomy and for women who have coronary artery disease or osteoporosis (American Geriatrics Society Clinical Practice Committee, 1997). Progestin should be added to prevent the development of endometrial cancer in women who did not have a hysterectomy unless frequent monitoring for the possible development of endometrial cancer is performed. It is possible, however, that the addition of progestin decreases the beneficial effect of estrogen on the brain. Hormone replacement therapy may increase slightly the incidence of breast cancer, which is a special concern in women with personal or family histories of breast cancer.

## FREE RADICAL SCAVENGERS

Although it is not known why nerve cells die in the brains of people with Alzheimer's disease, oxygen-derived free radicals may be involved (Beal, 1997). Free radicals are transient, highly reactive, toxic substances (because they have unpaired valence electrons) that are formed during normal metabolism in most tissues, including brain tissue. Free radicals may be involved in the toxic effect of β-amyloid and in the inflammatory response to brain cell death. Thus, cell death caused by β-amyloid protein or other toxic factors may lead to the increased formation of free radicals, which cause the death of additional brain cells.

The body has several defenses against free radicals, but, if the formation of free radicals is increased or the defenses are not effective, then cell damage can occur. One of the defensive mechanisms is provided by vitamin E, one of the free radical "scavengers"—compounds that react with and render harmless free radicals by forming paired valence electrons. Administering vitamin E to people with Alzheimer's disease delayed the loss of functional abilities, temporarily preserved independence in ADLs, and delayed institutionalization (Sano et al., 1997). A delay in the progression of dementia also was observed after administering ginkgo biloba extract, which also may prevent the toxic effects of free radicals (Oken, Storzbach, & Kaye, 1998). Use of these substances, however, requires further research to determine optimal dosage and drug combinations. When vitamin E was combined with selegiline, another medication that decreases free radical toxicity, the combination was less effective than either substance alone (Sano et al., 1997).

## ACETYLCHOLINESTERASE INHIBITORS

Another approach to slowing the progression of Alzheimer's disease involves the inhibition of acetylcholinesterase, an enzyme that breaks down acetylcholine. Acetylcholine is one of the substances (neurotransmitters) that nerve cells use to communicate with one another. It is released from the processes of one nerve cell and affects the function of neighboring cells. Alzheimer's disease causes a decrease in the number of nerve cells that make acetylcholine and, therefore, a loss of available acetylcholine. Because acetylcholine is necessary for normal memory function, this loss leads to memory impairment. Inhibiting acetylcholine destruction increases the effect of the remaining acetylcholine and improves memory and, possibly, other cognitive functions.

Several drugs that inhibit acetylcholinesterase have been developed. Two of them, tacrine (Cognex) and donepezil (Aricept), have been approved by the U.S. Food and Drug Administration for treatment of Alzheimer's disease, and others are in different stages of development. Donepezil has some advantages over tacrine: It does not produce liver damage, it is administered only once a day, and it does not require a gradual increase of the dose to reach full effect (Rogers et al., 1998). Donepezil has very few side effects, but it can produce stomach upset and sleeping difficulties. All cholinesterase inhibitors only delay the progression of the disease, and when they are stopped the person's condition declines to the stage of dementia that would most likely have been present had these drugs not been used. Tacrine was found to delay the progression of dementia by 6 months, but it may delay institutionalization by an even longer interval (Knopman et al., 1996).

> Mrs. Alba was prescribed donepezil and vitamin E therapy. The primary care physician weighed all of the risks and benefits of hormone replacement therapy. Because Mrs. Alba does not have a family history of breast cancer and stopped menstruating 6 years ago, estrogen replacement therapy was initiated. She is scheduled for frequent gynecological evaluations.

Several additional drugs for the treatment of Alzheimer's disease are in different stages of development. Some drugs act similarly to acetylcholine and others influence calcium movement through the nerve cell membrane. Other potential mechanisms that may be useful in the treatment of Alzheimer's disease include modification of β-amyloid and tau proteins and increased production of growth factors that protect nerve cells.

> About 2 weeks after the treatment was started, Mrs. Alba's memory gradually improved and she was able to resume her work as a waitress. Six months later, however, her memory problems returned and she eventually had to retire. Even though her dementia progressed, she retains a friendly attitude and appropriate social behaviors.

## INTERACTION BETWEEN DEMENTIA AND PERSONALITY

Many people with Alzheimer's disease retain vestiges of their personalities, even in moderate to severe stages of dementia. Individuals who were involved in social interactions throughout their lives (e.g., service personnel, salespeople) often retain the basic elements of social behavior, such as greetings, shaking hands, and giving compliments. Other individuals may develop one or more psychiatric symptoms that are described in other chapters in this book. There is some evidence that premorbid personality traits are related to subsequent psychiatric symptoms (Chatterjee et al., 1992). People who were neurotic and less assertive before developing dementia are likely to become depressed, whereas people who were hostile before developing dementia are likely to experience paranoid delusions. People who were neurotic and extroverted before developing dementia are likely to engage in aggressive behavior, whereas previous agreeableness decreases the probability of aggression (Van Cauter et al., 1998). The authors have found that some of the most difficult people to work with are former police officers. Former officers do not like being told what to do, and they use their experience in physical confrontation to prevent staff from providing personal care, which they perceive as an invasion of their privacy. Premorbid personality, however, is relatively inconsequential for adaptation of the person with Alzheimer's disease to a long-term care facility (Brandt et al., 1998).

## REFERENCES

Alzheimer's Disease and Related Dementia Guideline Panel. (1996). *Recognition and initial assessment of Alzheimer's disease and related dementias.* Rockville, MD: Agency for Health Care Policy and Research.

American College of Medical Genetics. (1995). Statement on use of apolipoprotein E testing in Alzheimer's disease. *Journal of the American Medical Association, 274,* 1627–1629.

American Geriatrics Society Clinical Practice Committee. (1997). Counseling postmenopausal women about preventive hormone therapy. *Journal of the American Geriatrics Society, 44,* 1120–1122.

American Psychiatric Association. (1994). *Diagnostic and statistical manual of mental disorders* (4th ed., pp. 123–133). Washington, DC: American Psychiatric Press.

Beal, M.F. (1997). Oxidative damage in neurodegenerative diseases. *Neuroscientist, 3,* 21–27.

Brandt, J., Campodonico, J.R., Rich, J.B., Baker, L., Steele, C., Ruff, T., Baker, A., & Lyketsos, C. (1998). Adjustment to residential placement in Alzheimer's disease patients: Does premorbid personality matter? *International Journal of Geriatric Psychiatry, 13,* 509–515.

Carlesimo, G.A., Mauri, M., Graceffa, A.M., Fadda, L., Loasses, A., Lorusso, S., & Caltagirone, C. (1998). Memory performances in young, elderly, and very old healthy individuals versus patients with Alzheimer's disease: Evidence for discontinuity between normal and pathological aging. *Journal of Clinical and Experimental Neuropsychology, 20,* 14–29.

Chatterjee, A., Strauss, M.E., Smyth, K.A., & Whitehouse, P.J. (1992). Personality changes in Alzheimer's disease. *Archives of Neurology, 49,* 486–491.

Corder, E.H., Saunders, A.M., Strittmatter, W.J., Schmechel, D.E., Gaskell, P.C., Small, G.W., Roses, A.D., Haines, J.L., & Pericak-Vance, M.A. (1993). Gene dose of apolipoprotein E type 4 allele and the risk of Alzheimer's disease in late onset families. *Science, 261,* 921–923.

Curran, M., Middleton, D., Edwardson, J., Perry, R., McKeith, I., Morris, C., & Neill, D. (1997). HLA-DR antigens associated with major genetic risk for late-onset Alzheimer's disease. *Neuroreport, 8,* 1467–1469.

Graves, A.B., Mortimer, J.A., Larson, E.B., Wenzlow, A., Bowen, J.D., & McCormick, W.C. (1996). Head circumference as a measure of cognitive reserve. Association with severity of impairment in Alzheimer's disease. *British Journal of Psychiatry, 169,* 86–92.

Kanai, M., Matsubara, E., Isoe, K., Urakami, K., Nakashima, K., Arai, H., Sasaki, H., Abe, K., Iwatsubo, T., Kosaka, T., Watanabe, M., Tomidokoro, Y., Shizuka, M., Mizushima, K., Nakamura, T., Igeta, Y., Ikeda, Y., Amari, M., Kawarabayashi, T., Ishiguro, K., Harigaya, Y., Wakabayashi, K., Okamoto, K., & Hirai, S. (1998). Longitudinal study of cerebrospinal fluid levels of tau, Ab1-40, and Ab1-42(43) in Alzheimer's disease: A study in Japan. *Annals of Neurology, 44,* 17–26.

Kertesz, A., Davidson, W., & Fox, H. (1997). Frontal behavioral inventory: Diagnostic criteria for frontal lobe dementia. *Canadian Journal of Neurological Sciences, 24,* 29–36.

Knopman, D., Schneider, L., Davis, K., Talwalker, S., Smith, F., Hoover, T., & Gracon, S. (1996). Long-term tacrine (Cognex) treatment: Effects on nursing home placement and mortality. *Neurology, 47,* 166–177.

Kolanowski, A.M., & Whall, A.L. (1996). Life-span perspective of personality in dementia. *Image: The Journal of Nursing Scholarship, 28,* 315–320.

Lee, P.N. (1994). Smoking and Alzheimer's disease: A review of the epidemiological evidence. *Neuroepidemiology, 13,* 131–144.

Levkoff, S.E., Evans, D., Liptzin, B., Cleary, P.D., Lipsitz, L.A., Wetle, T.T., Reilly, C.H., Pilgrim, D.M., Schor, J., & Rowe, J. (1992). Delirium: The occurrence and persistence of symptoms among elderly hospitalized patients. *Archives of Internal Medicine, 152,* 334–340.

Liao, A., Nitsch, R.M., Greenberg, S.M., Finckh, U., Blacker, D., Albert, M., Rebeck, G.W., Gomez-Isla, T., Clatworthy, A., Binetti, G., Hock, C., Mueller-Thomsen, T., Mann, U., Zuchowski, K., Beisiegel, U., Staehelin, H., Growdon, J.H., Tanzi, R.E., & Hyman, B.T. (1998). Genetic association of an α2-macroglobulin (Val1000Ile) polymorphism and Alzheimer's disease. *Human Molecular Genetics, 7,* 1953–1956.

Macdonald, A.J.D., & Treloar, A. (1996). Delirium and dementia: Are they distinct? *Journal of the American Geriatrics Society, 44,* 1001–1002.

Martyn, C.N., Coggon, D.N., Inskip, H., Lacey, R.F., & Young, W.F. (1997). Aluminum concentrations in drinking water and risk of Alzheimer's disease. *Epidemiology, 8,* 281–286.

Mayeux, R., Ottman, R., Maestre, G., Ngai, C., Tang, M.-X., Ginsberg, H., Chun, M., Tycko, B., & Shelanski, M. (1995). Synergistic effects of traumatic head injury and apolipoprotein-E4 in patients with Alzheimer's disease. *Neurology, 45,* 555–557.

McGeer, P.L., Schulzer, M., & McGeer, E.G. (1996). Arthritis and anti-inflammatory agents as possible protective factors for Alzheimer's disease: A review of 17 epidemiologic studies. *Neurology, 47,* 425–432.

McKeith, I.G., Fairbairn, A.F., Bothwell, R.A., Moore, P.B., Ferrier, I.N., Thompson, P., & Perry, R.H. (1994). An evaluation of the predictive validity and inter-rater reliability of clinical diagnostic criteria for senile dementia of Lewy body type. *Neurology, 44,* 872–877.

McKeith, I.G., Galasko, D., Kosaka, K., Perry, E.K., Dickson, D.W., Hansen, L.A., Salmon, D.P., Lowe, J., Mirra, S.S., Byrne, E.J., Lennox, G., Quinn, N.P., Edwardson,

J.A., Ince, P.G., Bergeron, C., Burns, A., Miller, B.L., Lovestone, S., Collerton, D., Jansen, E.N.H., Ballard, C., De Vos, R.A.I., Wilcock, G.K., & Jellinger, K.A. (1996). Consensus guidelines for the clinical and pathologic diagnosis of dementia with Lewy bodies (DLB): Report of the Consortium on DLB International Workshop. *Neurology, 47,* 1113–1124.

Mendez, M.F., Cherrier, M., Perryman, K.M., Pachana, N., Miller, B.L., & Cummings, J.L. (1996). Frontotemporal dementia versus Alzheimer's disease: Differential cognitive features. *Neurology, 47,* 1189–1194.

Mortimer, J.A., & Graves, A.B. (1993). Education and other socioeconomic determinants of dementia and Alzheimer's disease. *Neurology, 43*(Suppl. 4), S39–S44.

Mulnard, R.A., Cotman, C.W., Kawas, C., van Dyck, C.H., Sano, M., Doody, R., Koss, E., Pfeiffer, E., Jin, S., Gamst, A., Grundman, M., Thomas, R., & Thal, L.J. (2000). Estrogen replacement therapy for treatment of mild to moderate Alzheimer's disease: A randomized controlled trial. *Journal of the American Medical Association, 283,* 1007–1015.

Oken, B.S., Storzbach, D.M., & Kaye, J.A. (1998). The efficacy of *Ginkgo biloba* on cognitive function in Alzheimer's disease. *Archives of Neurology, 55,* 1409–1415.

Paganini-Hill, A., & Henderson, V.W. (1996). Estrogen replacement therapy and risk of Alzheimer's disease. *Archives of Internal Medicine, 156,* 2213–2217.

Pericak-Vance, M.A., Bass, M.P., Yamaoka, L.H., Gaskell, P.C., Scott, W.K., Terwedow, H.A., Menold, M.M., Conneally, P.M., Small, G.W., Vance, J.M., Saunders, A.M., Roses, A.D., & Haines, J.L. (1997). Complete genomic screen in late-onset familial Alzheimer's disease. Evidence for a new locus on chromosome 12. *Journal of the American Medical Association, 278,* 1237–1241.

Raby, C.A., Morganti-Kossmann, M.C., Kossmann, T., Stahel, P.F., Watson, M.D., Evans, L.M., Mehta, P.D., Spiegel, K., Kuo, Y.M., Roher, A.E., & Emmerling, M.R. (1998). Traumatic brain injury increases β-amyloid peptide 1-42 in cerebrospinal fluid. *Journal of Neurochemistry, 71,* 2505–2509.

Reifler, B.V. (1997). Pre-dementia. *Journal of the American Geriatrics Society, 45,* 776–777.

Rogers, S.L., Farlow, M.R., Doody, R.S., Mohs, R., Friedhoff, L.T., & and the Donepezil Study Group. (1998). A 24 week, double blind, placebo-controlled trial of donepezil in patients with Alzheimer's disease. *Neurology, 50,* 136–145.

Sano, M., Ernesto, C., Thomas, R.G., Klauber, M.R., Schafer, K., Grundman, M., Woodbury, P., Growdon, J., Cotman, D.W., Pfeiffer, E., Schneider, L.S., & Thal, L.J. (1997). A controlled trial of selegiline, alpha-tocopherol, or both as treatment for Alzheimer's disease. *New England Journal of Medicine, 336,* 1216–1222.

Snowdon, D.A. (1997). Aging and Alzheimer's disease: Lessons from the Nun Study. *Gerontologist, 37,* 150–156.

Snowdon, D.A., Greiner, L.H., Mortimer, J.A., Riley, K.P., Greiner, P.A., & Markesbery, W.R. (1997). Brain infarction and the clinical expression of Alzheimer's disease: The nun study. *Journal of the American Medical Association, 277,* 813–817.

Snowdon, D.A., Kemper, S.J., Mortimer, J.A., Greiner, L.H., Wekstein, D.R., & Markesbery, W.R. (1996). Linguistic ability in early life and cognitive function and Alzheimer's disease in late life: Findings from the nun study. *Journal of the American Medical Association, 275,* 528–532.

Tilley, L., Morgan, K., & Kalsheker, N. (1998). Genetic risk factors in Alzheimer's disease. *Journal of Clinical Pathology: Molecular Pathology, 51*, 293–304.

Treloar, A.J., & Macdonald, A.J. (1997a). Outcome of delirium: I. Outcome of delirium diagnosed by DSM III-R, ICD-10, and Camdex and derivation of the Reversible Cognitive Dysfunction Scale among acute geriatric inpatients. *International Journal of Geriatric Psychiatry, 12*, 609–613.

Treloar, A.J., & Macdonald, A.J. (1997b). Outcome of delirium: II. Clinical features of reversible cognitive dysfunction—are they the same as accepted definitions of delirium? *International Journal of Geriatric Psychiatry, 12*, 614–618.

Van Cauter, E., Moreno-Reyes, R., Akseki, E., L'Hermite-Balériaux, M., Hirschfeld, U., Leproult, R., & Copinschi, G. (1998). Rapid phase advance of the 24-h melatonin profile in response to afternoon dark exposure. *American Journal of Physiology, 275*, E47–E54.

Vasterling, J.J., Seltzer, B., Foss, J.W., & Vanderbrook, V. (1995). Unawareness of deficit in Alzheimer's disease: Domain-specific differences and disease correlates. *Neuropsychiatry, Neuropsychology, and Behavioral Neurology, 8*, 26–32.

Verhey, F.R.J., Lodder, J., Rozendaal, N., & Jolles, J. (1996). Comparison of seven sets of criteria used for the diagnosis of vascular dementia. *Neuroepidemiology, 15*, 166–172.

Yaffe, K., Sawaya, G., Lieberburg, I., & Grady, D. (1998). Estrogen therapy in postmenopausal women: Effects on cognitive function and dementia. *Journal of the American Medical Association, 279*, 688–695.

# 2

# Functional Impairment

Functional impairment has both cognitive and physical components. When cognitive deficits are severe enough to interfere with functioning, the criteria for the diagnosis of dementia are met (American Psychiatric Association, 1994). Physical impairments may be the result of dementia, comorbidities, or disuse. Progressive cognitive and physical decline increases the inability of people with dementia to cope with either environmental or internal stressors (Hall & Buckwalter, 1987). According to the model of behavioral symptoms of dementia presented in the Introduction, functional impairments lead to dependence in activities of daily living (ADLs), the inability to initiate meaningful activities, and other behavioral symptoms. Because functional impairment is a primary consequence of dementia, the model suggests that preventing, improving, or supporting functional ability will have a positive effect on multiple behavioral consequences of dementia.

Barbara Browne is a 74-year-old woman living in the suburbs with her husband of more than 50 years. They have a close, loving relationship. Since retiring 9 years ago from the telephone company, where she worked as an operator, she has enjoyed cooking, knitting, and sewing children's clothing for charitable donations. She also enjoys taking walks and playing board games with her husband. Both enjoy traveling and visiting their children and grandchildren, who live nearby. In addition to her roles as wife, mother, and grandmother, Mrs. Browne is active in church and neighborhood activities.

During the past several months, Mrs. Browne's family has noticed subtle changes in her functional abilities. Her husband reports that she plans a meal, but then spends hours unsuccessfully trying to find a particular recipe, and she ends up crying when there is no meal to eat at 7:00 P.M. As they packed to leave for vacation, she was unable to find their traveler's checks or the addresses of friends to visit and postcards to send. She became short-tempered with Mr. Browne, telling him, "You must have taken them because I know I put them right here!" Mrs. Browne's children observe that Mr. Browne commonly fills in words and finishes sentences for his wife during a conversation, reminds her about the topic of conversation, or stops her when she repeats a question that has already been raised and answered, often several times.

## COGNITIVE IMPAIRMENT

Cognitive deficits in dementia occur in several spheres, including memory impairment, aphasia, apraxia, agnosia, and disturbance in executive function (American Psychiatric Association, 1994; Klein & Kowall, 1998). These impairments limit a person's ability to engage in activities required or desired for independent functioning and quality of life (Volicer, Hurley, & Camberg, 1999). According to Lawton (1995), there is a hierarchy of cognitive competence, ranging from complex functions (e.g., creative innovation, problem solving) to simple aspects (e.g., perception, sensory reception). As dementia progresses, cognitive skills accessible by the person also decline, with complex functions affected first. At the same time, interventions matched to the person's functional level can maintain optimal function, increase involvement with the environment, and enhance a sense of autonomy (Burgener, 1998).

### ASSESSMENT OF COGNITIVE FUNCTION

One standard measure of cognitive function is the Mini-Mental Status Examination (MMSE; Folstein, Folstein, & McHugh, 1975). The advantages of the MMSE are that it is short, it is easy to administer, it is a standardized instrument used across all care settings and familiar to most professional caregivers, and it examines a wide range of cognitive functions. Therefore, the MMSE score, which ranges from 0 (complete impairment) to 30 (no impairment), describes the extent of cognitive impairment and communicates this level to others. For example, the following information was recorded on Mrs. Browne's outpatient medical record:

Mrs. Browne has a short-term memory deficit, but her long-term memory is preserved. She thinks the year is 1955. Her attention span is severely impaired. She is unable to perform a three-step command, but she can follow directions one at a time with visual and verbal cues.

This information should be used to match Mrs. Browne's care plan with her cognitive ability. For example, the fact that she could follow simple directions with cues is a guide to the kind of help that she will need with ADLs (see Chapter 5). Her preserved long-term memory can be used with reminiscence therapy (see Chapters 6 and 7).

As the dementia progresses, the MMSE score ultimately becomes 0 and the test is no longer able to differentiate levels of cognitive functioning. For this reason, the Bedford Alzheimer Nursing Severity Scale (BANS-S; Volicer, Hurley, Lathi, & Kowall, 1994) was developed. The BANS-S assesses functional capacity, even in severe dementia, by combining ratings of cognitive (e.g., speech, eye contact) and functional (e.g., dressing, eating, ambulating) deficits with the occurrence of pathological symptoms (e.g., sleep-wake cycle disturbance, muscle rigidity/contractures). BANS-S scores range from 7 (no impairment) to 28 (complete impairment).

## SHORT-TERM MEMORY LOSS

Short-term memory loss, caused by neuropathological changes in the brain, is characterized by difficulty recalling recent events and learning new material (Klein & Kowall, 1998). Other factors also may contribute to short-term memory loss. For example, attentional deficits prevent the person from focusing on one thing long enough for it to become transcribed into memory. Difficulty paying attention is particularly noticeable if multiple stimuli are occurring simultaneously. The diseased brain cannot select the most important stimulus and ignore all others, but rather gives each stimulus equal attention or randomly jumps from one stimulus to another.

Mrs. Browne shows several signs of short-term memory impairment. She is unable to find things (recipes, addresses) and does not remember the topic of a conversation, both during and after it has occurred. The extent to which she is aware of her short-term memory problem varies, as does her reaction. Sometimes she becomes frustrated, for example, when she tried unsuccessfully to find a recipe. At other times she blames others, as she did with the "missing" address book. At still other times, she does not seem to be aware that she has forgotten, as when her husband reminds her of the topic of the conversation in which she is participating. These responses are common and create a challenge for the caregiver, who is in the position of helping to correct the deficit or filling in the blanks and who never knows what reaction to expect from the person with dementia. Families need information and support to cope with these fluctuations. The health care provider also can recommend the use of a journal in which the family can record such things as "good topics"—those that spark interest or enjoyment, favorite memories that can be used for reminiscence, or situations that lead to better functioning. The family also should record "bad topics" that may have stimulated decreased functioning, increased awareness of the problem, or a negative reaction. During outpatient visits, the care provider can review these entries and help the family identify behavior patterns that they can use in planning their care for the person with dementia.

Assessment of memory is a sensitive topic. Although the assessment provides information that is important for identifying the extent of the problem, evaluating changes, and planning care, the memory assessment can be embarrassing or frustrating and anxiety-producing for the older person who is aware of performance difficulties. Great sensitivity is required to put the person at ease and to acknowledge feelings generated by this experience. The assessment can be done yearly or when there is an acute change in the person's behavior. More frequent questioning or insistence that the person remember, as one would do in reality orientation, should be avoided.

## EXECUTIVE FUNCTIONS

Executive functions, such as problem solving and judgment, require the ability to think abstractly and make connections among relevant facts, as well as the ability to generate logical alternatives in problem situations (Quayhagen, Quayhagen, Corbeil, Roth, & Rodgers, 1995). These cognitive functions depend on the frontal lobes and association areas of the frontal, parietal, and temporal cerebral cortices. The time that Mrs. Browne spent an entire day searching unsuccessfully for a missing recipe and ended up crying and without dinner is an example of this impairment. Other common examples include wearing a coat and gloves on a hot summer day and insisting on driving even after repeated accidents and episodes of getting lost (see Chapter 8).

## APHASIA

Mrs. Browne rarely leaves her husband's side. Today, their children have come to have lunch with Mrs. Browne so that Mr. Browne can have a much-needed break to go out with some friends. She asks, "Where's Dad?" every few minutes. Although the Browne children noticed that their father filled in words for their mother during conversations, they had not realized, until he was not there to help, that she had trouble finding the words she was looking for. Their father had been so graceful and unobtrusive in supporting his wife that the family had no idea of the scope of her disability. For example, while telling her daughters, Beth and Betsy, that she had been to a funeral, Mrs. Browne says, "Oh, you should have ... oh, it was so ... at the church, so many people, just beautiful with all those ... give me a minute to collect my thoughts, ... oh, you should have seen. Where's your father? Dad, tell the girls ... oh, you should have seen ... ." When he returns, Mr. Browne asks his wife if she wants him to describe where they had been and she says "yes." When he says they had been to a funeral, Mrs. Browne not only agrees but she also tries to add to the story. "You won't believe who we saw!" she says. "Dad, tell them." She becomes impatient when he does not name the "right" person. Finally, she says, "I can't tell you right now."

Aphasia is the loss of the ability to use symbols to communicate. Expressive aphasia is the inability to form words or express oneself clearly orally or in writing. Receptive aphasia refers to the decreased ability to understand spoken or written language (Stehman, Strachan, Glenner, Glenner, & Neubauer, 1996). Mrs. Browne, who is at an early stage of dementia, has trouble finding words, especially nouns. Her speech is fluent but lacking in content. She uses circumlocution, talking around the word she cannot find. In fact, this can be an effective strategy in communicating and can be a way to cover the deficit. Mrs. Browne is aware that she cannot find the words she wants, and it is a source of embarrassment and frustration to her. Her husband demonstrates respect for her by asking if she wants help. His comments serve as cues, enabling her to again participate in conversation. It is important to continue to talk with the person who has dementia, who continues to have a need for participation and understanding (Bohling, 1991; Silverio & Koenig-Coste, 1999). Guidelines for communicating for the person who has dementia (Silverio & Koenig-Coste, 1999) and for the caregiver (Benjamin, 1999; Burgener, Jirovec, Murrell, & Barton, 1992; Raia, 1999) are listed as follows:

### For the person with dementia

Try not to be embarrassed when you cannot find the right words.

Speak slowly; ask for help from your family when you cannot think of what you want to say.

Do not be embarrassed to ask people to repeat themselves.

Share your feelings with a friend, family member, clergy, or counselor. It is okay to feel angry, sad, or frustrated.

### For the caregiver of the person with dementia

Provide opportunities for meaningful communication.

Use a validating approach; people with dementia respond to nonverbal cues.

Nonverbal cues include smiles, a calm demeanor, and sensitive listening.
Enter the reality of the person with dementia.
Acknowledge underlying emotions to make the person feel loved and safe.
Use communication to provide purpose and direction.

Difficulty with verbal communication is paralleled by similar problems with reading and writing. Mrs. Browne will have the same problem with word finding if she tries to write. If she has difficulty understanding spoken words, then she will likewise be unable to understand what she reads. Although a person may still "read" the newspaper out of habit, he or she will not be able to recount what is read. Nevertheless, it is important to keep the person engaged with the world by including him or her in conversation about familiar topics, avoiding any pressure to perform, and allowing the person to continue with patterns that convey a sense of security. Reminiscence about meaningful experiences from the past, which may be remembered longer because they are stored in long-term memory, can facilitate meaningful communication even when the person is no longer able to initiate speech independently (Kovach & Henschel, 1996). Likewise, favorite music can provide a means of communication as well as relaxation (see Chapters 6 and 7). Often, people with dementia can sing familiar songs such as "Happy Birthday to You" or recite overlearned verses even when they cannot initiate speech.

When comprehension of language is impaired, television can be a source of confusion and even fear, and it should be avoided. Some possible exceptions include sports events or musical programs, if the person with mild or moderately severe dementia seems to enjoy them. These exceptions should be determined on an individual basis and reevaluated at regular intervals.

Beth and Betsy confide in each other that they hate to call their parents at night because their mother "can't even get a sentence out" and it is "too painful to hear her like this." At a family gathering filled with noise and excitement, it was even worse. Mrs. Browne felt uneasy so she drank a few martinis to relax. Her speech became devoid of content and peppered with word substitutions (*paraphrasias;* e.g., "needle" when she meant "noodle") and made-up words (*neologisms;* e.g., "moombas"). She confused the names of her grandchildren and finally resorted to calling them "whatever your name is" (*circumlocution*). Some of the children found this amusing, whereas others' feelings were hurt ("Nana can't even remember who I am!"). When Mrs. Browne is unable to identify objects by name, she uses phrases such as "whatchamacallit" or "thingamajig," or says, "You know what I mean."

Fatigue, activities out of the routine, alcohol, and a high-stimulus environment are stressors that increase functional impairment as well as secondary consequences such as anxiety (see Chapter 7) or agitation (see Chapter 12). Mrs. Browne's aphasia is exaggerated by each of these factors individually and cumulatively. Because the person with dementia becomes more dependent on the environment as the disease progresses (Lawton, 1982), the environment needs to be adapted to facilitate the individual's functioning (in this case, communication). Strategies that the Browne family should try include visiting early in the day, after a rest, or at whatever time of day Mrs. Browne is at her best; limiting visitors to a few at a time; and substituting caffeine-free herbal tea for alcohol. Having a quiet place where Mrs. Browne can be with her grandchildren individually, combined with cueing, can be an effective strategy. For example, Beth might bring her daughter and say, "Mom, Bridget wants to show you the picture she drew." This kind of approach takes the pressure off Mrs. Browne to remember her granddaughter's name, and the child's picture serves as a prop for both grandmother and granddaughter to communicate.

Other interventions to facilitate communication are cueing, reminiscence, favorite familiar music, environmental modification, and stimulus control. The health care provider can supply resources to families to help them understand what the person with dementia is going through and to help their children understand why a grandparent forgets their names. (Several wonderful books have been written specifically for children, including *Nanny's Special Gift* [Potatacke, 1993] and *I Remember! Cried Grandma Pinky* [Wahl, 1994]. The Alzheimer's Association [1998] has compiled an extensive bibliography of Alzheimer's disease information for children and adolescents, including books, articles, and videos.)

As the dementia progresses, a person's other expressive and receptive language functions are lost. The person may mumble incoherently or groan (vocalization) but not speak (verbalization). Ultimately, the person may become mute. In every case it is still important to talk to the person. The fact that a person cannot speak does not mean that he or she cannot hear or understand nonverbal communication. Even when verbal language is lost, nonverbal communication by way of tone of voice, smiles, and body language may be comforting.

Assessment of aphasia provides caregivers with a baseline from which to monitor changes. Perhaps more important, communication can be geared to the degree of impairment and the nature of remaining abilities. The goals are to support a person's remaining language skills and maintain his or her connection to the outside world throughout the progression of the dementia. A speech assessment tool that was developed specifically for people with advanced dementia (Volicer et al., 1987) includes the assessment of spontaneous speech, comprehension, naming, and repetition.

## APRAXIA

Mrs. Browne was not able to complete the three-step command from the MMSE. In fact, it seemed as though she did not even try to do anything she was asked during her visit to the clinic. Staff are quite sure that she understands simple directions, and they know that she is physically able to do what they ask. After all, they saw her walk in, take off her coat and hang it up, and pick up a magazine from the table. Why, then, would she not get on the scale when they told her they had to weigh her and asked her to step up? Mr. Browne reported that his wife dressed herself if they chose her clothes together, but when staff asked her to change into an examining gown, she just sat there. She did not even lift her foot when they asked to remove her shoes. They had to lift her foot for her, at which point she kicked off her own shoe.

Apraxia is the inability to initiate complex learned motor movements (Stehman et al., 1996). The person with apraxia may be able to perform an activity spontaneously but not be able to do the same activity on command. Apraxia is the reason why Mrs. Browne is able to dress herself at home, out of habit and in response to seeing her clothes, but is not able to undress on command in the clinic. As the dementia progresses to a more advanced stage, the person may be able to imitate an activity, even when unable to initiate it, or he or she may be able to respond to visual cues better than to verbal directions alone. For example, although Mrs. Browne may be unable to follow a command such as "wash your face," she still may be able to wash her face if handed a washcloth, or continue an activity, such as eating, once someone helps her to get started.

Apraxia results from a breakdown in the pathways in the brain between where an idea for action occurs or a direction is understood and where it is carried out. Problems with sequencing also occur, so the person may not know what to do first or what to do next. There are several specific kinds of apraxia. All refer to the same basic pathological process applied to different skills, for example, dressing, chewing (mastication), writing (graphomotor), and speaking. Spontaneous activity may be possible when an on-command activity is not possible because a different pathway, which depends more on habit than on planning, is used. Visual cues or helping the person get started likewise may circumvent the disrupted path. The more complex the task, the greater the person's problem with figuring out how to begin and how to proceed, and the greater the potential for the person with dementia to fail to execute the task, feel frustrated and stressed, and, ultimately, be stimulated into experiencing a catastrophic reaction. Therefore, an effective intervention for both promoting functional performance and preventing behavior problems is to break complex tasks such as bathing or dressing into step-by-step segments that can be completed one at a time. This is discussed in detail in Chapter 5.

Understanding apraxia is critical to avoid attributing the person's behavior to "lack of motivation" or "being obstinate." Apraxia is a motor-planning problem. The behaviors that are demonstrated by Mrs. Browne are typical. Caregivers must be able to identify apraxia and differentiate it from depression (Chapter 3), anxiety (Chapter 7), or resistiveness to care (Chapter 9) to match interventions with the cause of the problems. A referral to an occupational therapist may be useful in this regard.

## AGNOSIA

As part of her neuropsychological assessment, Mrs. Browne is asked to name common objects. When shown a pencil, she says, "pretzel," and when shown a watch, she says, "tick, tock, arm, what time." When she is shown a comb, she says nothing, and when the comb is handed to her and she is asked to show how it is used, she begins to brush her teeth. The neuropsychologist explains to Mr. Browne that the problem with naming (*anomia*) is part of aphasia, while lack of recognition of what the comb is for is called *agnosia*.

Agnosia is the inability to recognize familiar objects by sight, touch, taste, smell, or sound. The most striking example is the famous case study that forms Oliver Sacks's 1985 book *The Man Who Mistook His Wife for a Hat*. The patient had a severe case of agnosia that was caused by damage to the association areas of the cerebral hemispheres. He had lost the ability to recognize even his own wife, whom he did, indeed, mistake for a hat. The book chronicles the frustration and difficulty of living with agnosia. Mrs. Browne presents a somewhat confusing picture at first glance. Clearly, she knows how a watch is used, and resorts to circumlocution when she cannot find the word "watch." This is an example of aphasia rather than agnosia. The substitution of "pretzel" for "pencil" is equivocal; this may be a case of substituting one word for another (paraphrasia), or it may be agnosia. One way to clarify the difference is to observe whether she uses the pencil to write. The example of the comb is a clear indication of agnosia. Agnosia causes functional impairment and also can present a safety hazard if a person puts inedible things in his or her mouth, pours water into a toaster, or puts silverware into his or her socks. People with dementia may not recognize the bathroom or remember how to use the toilet. Signs or a picture on the door, which may have been useful during the early stages of dementia, lose their effectiveness when the person with agnosia loses the ability to recognize the picture and associate it with the use of the bathroom.

Agnosia also may explain people's fear of entering an institutional bathroom. They do not recognize the purpose of this steel, porcelain, and tile room with its hydraulic furniture for lifting people and whirring motors for whirlpool baths. This lack of recognition can result in anxiety, resistiveness, and other behavioral symptoms as shown in the model of behavioral symptoms of dementia that was described in the Introduction. Environmental modifications (described in Chapters 8 and 13) help to compensate for the effects of agnosia.

Interesting research is being done to understand how people with dementia interpret facial expressions. When facial expressions, such as joy, anger, and boredom, are not recognized, this form of agnosia can cause misinterpretation. Because people respond according to their perceptions, reactions that seem bizarre or even aggressive to people who do not have dementia may make perfect sense to the person with dementia.

## INTERVENTION STRATEGIES
## FOR THE PERSON WITH COGNITIVE IMPAIRMENT

Interventions for the person with cognitive impairment should be geared toward creating an environment in which the person can experience positive emotions and preventing excess disability, which may be induced either by expecting too much or by expecting too little from the person. Caregivers should avoid frustrating the person by asking questions that he or she cannot answer (Gerdner, Hall, & Buckwalter, 1996) or demanding that he or she remember ("I just told you!"). Patience and respect must characterize every encounter. Raia (1999) described the concept of habilitation as "therapeutic intervention [that] supports the person's remaining cognitive capacities, respects his or her adult needs, and emphasizes meaningful activity" (p. 23).

Understanding the cause of the problem should direct solutions and identify specific interventions. For example, if the functional consequences of agnosia and apraxia decrease self-care independence in an activity, the caregiver should use multiple "channels" to overcome the deficit. To maintain Mrs. Browne's independence in toothbrushing, the caregiver could say, "Here is your toothbrush. You can brush your teeth. Smell the mint in the toothpaste. What a beautiful color blue. Do you want to taste it?" The caregiver then might show his or her own teeth and point to Mrs. Browne's mouth. If Mrs. Browne does not then take the toothbrush and begin brushing because of apraxia, then she may need help getting started. The caregiver should put the brush in Mrs. Browne's hand and cover Mrs. Browne's hand as a guide and bring it to her mouth to initiate the procedure for her to continue on her own. Other strategies are recommended according to the stage of dementia that the person is in.

## Mild to Moderate Stages

Memory aids, such as calendars and notes, may be helpful in the early stages of dementia, but their usefulness fades when the person can no longer remember to use them or what they mean. Cueing and creating connections to familiar things and simplifying and breaking down tasks into small parts that the person can complete one by one are useful (Beck et al., 1997). Group interactions, structured recreational activities, and reminiscence therapy can facilitate cognitive functioning at these early stages (Burgener, 1998).

Practice is a positive way to help the person with dementia maintain cognitive skills longer. Quayhagen and colleagues (1995) developed a cognitive remediation program for use by caregivers of people with dementia living at home and tested its effects on outcomes of cognitive functioning and behavior. Exercises included word fluency, immediate and long-term verbal and nonverbal recall and recognition, and problem solving. Every exercise required active participation by the care recipient. People in the experimental group improved in cognitive function and had fewer behavior problems, whereas those in the control group continued to decline in cognitive function. The program required sustained energy on the part of caregivers. Nonetheless, the results add to a growing body of evidence that procedural learning can and does occur in people with dementia and that the rate of decline in function can be slowed by the prevention of excess disability.

## Moderate to Severe Stages

Long-term memory is retained longer than recent memory. Burgener (1998) observed that people retain skills and knowledge from their past, even in advanced stages of dementia. She recommended assessing their previous abilities and focusing on their retained abilities and encouraged maintaining consistent structured routines to facilitate involvement and decrease frustration by promoting familiarity. An interesting example is Greiner et al.'s (1997) study of people with dementia playing dominoes; the subjects were skilled players before they developed dementia. The researchers found that when gamelike situations were created, people with dementia remained skilled at playing, even though they failed explicit memory tests for information related to their skills. The same phenomenon has been observed for language and musical skills. Greiner and colleagues suggested that implicit memory allows the selective use of preserved skills—the knowledge is intact but is accessible only in particular contexts. The clinical relevance of this "implicit memory" is supported by clinical evidence that reminiscence and music can be used to access retained memory.

## PHYSICAL IMPAIRMENT

Physical function is affected by the dementing process itself and by the presence of immobility or comorbidity. Each of these factors has both independent and additive effects, and each merits both a preventive and a restorative care plan. In addition, many of the medications that are commonly prescribed for people with dementia affect mobility either directly or indirectly.

### DEMENTIA

Physical impairment may be directly related to dementia according to brain pathology. For example, the progressive cortical, extrapyramidal, and pyramidal systems dysfunction of dementia causes neuromotor changes that result in declining function (Franssen, Kluger, Torossian, & Reisberg, 1993; Souren, Franssen, & Reisberg, 1997). For the person with vascular or ischemic dementia, the infarcts may have caused weakness of an extremity, exaggerated deep tendon reflexes, or gait abnormalities, in addition to the cognitive effects. People with diffuse Lewy body disease may exhibit parkinsonian symptoms that affect posture, balance, and gait. Alzheimer's disease causes physical impairment by affecting a person's ability to perform complex learned tasks that are required to carry out ADLs. Agnosia can cause a person to be unable to recognize and react safely to objects in his or her path, contributing to falls. *Paratonia,* an involuntary rigidity response, causes a flexed posture, loss of balance, and falls. Alzheimer's disease may result in abnormal reflexes, seizures, myoclonic jerks, and rigidity in the later stages of the disease. Because of progressive cerebral pathology, people lose the ability to walk and then the ability to stand; this results in immobility (Klein & Kowall, 1998; Trudeau, 1999; Volicer, Hurley, & Mahoney, 1995). Although the neurological changes are progressive, Trudeau (1999) cautioned against giving "too much power to the disease" by attributing all physical impairment to the dementing process. Both immobility and comorbidity are treatable risk factors for physical impairment that also guide assessment and intervention.

### IMMOBILITY

Losses of muscle mass, strength, and flexibility have been linked to immobility, and these risk factors are magnified when physical restraints are used (Trudeau, 1999). In addition, deconditioning and loss of endurance result from disuse, causing decreased activity tolerance as a result of fatigability and further contributing to generalized weakness. Prolonged sitting or bed rest can result in leg contractures, which make walking difficult or impossible. Many commonly used medications predispose individuals to decreased mobility by causing sedation, impaired balance, and altered muscle tone (Stone, Wyman,

& Salisbury, 1999). The hazards of immobility, when combined with neuro-motor deterioration, compound the chances that people with dementia will be injured at some point.

## COMORBIDITY

Mrs. Browne is physically healthy, except for the presence of osteoporo-sis and spinal stenosis, which cause her severe leg pain, especially at night. She was referred to physical therapy for evaluation, but she fell and fractured a hip before her appointment. Mr. Browne already had been questioning his ability to manage his wife's care and worries about her welfare if something should happen to him. A plan is created to admit Mrs. Browne to a nursing facility following her discharge from the hospital.

Physical impairment also can be caused by other health problems. Dementia is primarily a disease of older adults. Although age itself does not cause physical impairment, the frequency of physical impairments does increase as a person grows older. Older people with dementia have the same risks as do all older adults for health conditions that impair physical function (e.g., cardiovascular disease, osteoarthritis, undernutrition, polypharmacy). Other common symptoms (e.g., pain, sleep disturbance), may contribute to an impairment in physical function (Leidy, 1994). Acute changes in physical function usually are the result of an acute event such as a cerebrovascular acci-dent, a hip fracture, or an intercurrent infection.

## INTERVENTION STRATEGIES FOR PHYSICAL IMPAIRMENT

The goals of intervention strategies for the person with physical impairment are to maintain the highest level of functional capacity for as long as possible and to restore capacity that may be remediable. General guidelines are to

- Prevent excess disability (e.g., assisted ambulation versus bed rest to pre-vent immobility)
- Treat other conditions that lead to physical decline (e.g., pain that interferes with walking)
- Identify and respond rapidly to acute changes in function (e.g., early diag-nosis of infection)
- Adapt care to the neuromotor changes that accompany the progression of the dementia

## Mild to Moderate Stages

A planned program of physical activity benefits all older adults. Current activity recommendations from the National Institutes of Health for cardiovascular health include 30 minutes or more (cumulative) of moderate-intensity activity every day (Jones & Jones, 1997). Resistive exercises improve strength and balance and decrease falls in older adults (Fiatarone et al., 1993; Tideiksaar, 1998). Many people with dementia exhibit a need for movement, which should be encouraged. Some people actually become more physically fit because pacing is a form of exercise. Exercising, such as walking or dancing, is among the pleasant activities that have been identified for people with dementia (Logsdon & Teri, 1997; see also Chapter 6). Walking programs improve physical function, mood, and communication; promote engagement with the environment; and decrease daytime sleeping and agitated behaviors (Trudeau, 1999).

These programs provide planned, supervised activity on a regular basis and comply with the intent of the Nursing Home Reform Act as specified in the Omnibus Budget Reconciliation Act of 1987 (OBRA '87). One of the standards of care requirements of this act specifies "that persons receive the necessary care and services to attain or maintain the highest practicable physical, mental and psychosocial well-being, in accordance with the comprehensive assessment and plan of care" (p. 395). In both community and institutional long-term care settings adequate time and assistance in a supportive environment must be provided to meet this standard.

Trudeau (1999) recommended evaluating whether changes in physical function are acute (less than 1 month) or long-standing. People who experience acute decline in physical function in general have the potential for rehabilitation. An interdisciplinary team including experts in nursing, medicine, pharmacy, physical therapy, and occupational therapy is necessary to assess people's functional impairment from multiple perspectives and to plan and carry out coordinated interventions to meet the goals of prevention and restoration. In a study of a general population of long-term care residents, Morris and colleagues (1998) found that people with recent improvement in physical function are at risk for subsequent decline if their newly acquired functional ability is not supported. Planned rehabilitation to sustain gains is needed.

When considering rehabilitation for people with dementia, it is important to weigh carefully the burdens as well as the benefits to them. This issue has been explored in relation to the use of restraints (Rader, 1995), but it can be applied to any intervention. On the one hand, it is clear that rehabilitation potential exists and that people with dementia can benefit from interventions that are designed to maximize function, which also may improve their quality of life. On the other hand, rehabilitation is limited by the ability of an individual to follow directions and remember instructions. Rehabilitation also may become counterproductive if it leads to discomfort and fatigue (Trudeau, 1999; Volicer et al., 1998). Still, the expertise of rehabilitation staff can be called on to evaluate the usefulness of assistive devices and to help create a positive and supportive environment for people with dementia.

## Moderate to Severe Stages

As neuromotor deterioration progresses, caregivers must adapt interventions and the environment to compensate for changes in muscle tone and reflexes that affect a person's posture, balance, range of motion, and ability to cooperate with care (Souren et al., 1997; Trudeau, 1999). Falling is most likely to occur when the person is turning, backing up, reaching for an object, getting out of a chair, or attempting to move unassisted from one location to another (Stone et al., 1999). A preventive program should be instituted that employs the expertise of an interdisciplinary team to assess mobility, prevent falls, promote proper positioning, and implement environmental adaptations, such as redesigning furniture or introducing appropriate assistive devices (Trudeau, 1999).

The Merry Walker (Merry Walker Corp., Richmond, Iowa) is a steel-constructed walker on four wheels that allows people to maintain mobility in an upright position with modified independence (Trudeau, 1999). This walker includes a built-in seat located behind the individual that enhances safety by limiting falls and compensates for decreased endurance by allowing the person to sit down when he or she becomes fatigued (see Chapter 6). The effect of using the Merry Walker on the quality of life of people with severe dementia is being studied, and preliminary data are quite promising.

## Terminal Stage

Special positioning to support a person's trunk and limbs may be necessary in the late stages of dementia because paratonia results in a generally flexed posture and labile balance and contributes to the development of contractures. This involuntary rigidity response to passive movement is intermittent and may recede suddenly, only to resume moments later (Trudeau, 1999). Slow, gentle range-of-motion exercises for 10 minutes four times a day help a person maintain his or her full range of motion, delay rigidity, and prevent contractures (Stone et al., 1999). Safety precautions, such as padded siderails on the bed, are used to protect the person who develops myoclonic jerks or seizures during the terminal stage. The environment must be free of small objects that could cause choking if swallowed.

Caregiver education about the effects of neuromotor deterioration on the person's ability to cooperate during caregiving activities is important to promote understanding and effective care. For example, return of the primitive grasp reflex can result in the person exhibiting the behavior of grabbing and not letting go. Giving the person something to hold during caregiving, such as a towel or a colorful geometric-shaped object, helps to prevent him or her from grabbing the caregiver. When grabbing does occur, a gentle stroking of the back of the person's hand is more effective than trying to pull away or pry the person's fingers open; these actions serve only to further stimulate the reflex. Paratonic rigidity, also called *gegenhalten,* causes an involuntary motor response that is equal in force but opposite in direction to movement that is initiated by the caregiver. This phenomenon can precipitate behaviors such as adduction that make caregiving difficult (see also Chapter 9). Understanding the neuromotor etiology prevents informed caregivers from blaming the person. Gentle, slow movements should be used to prevent the rigidity response. Because rigidity waxes and wanes, an alternative for the caregiver is to pause for a short time before resuming the movement that initiated the response.

## REFERENCES

Alzheimer's Association. (1998). *A selected list of resources: Alzheimer's information for children and adolescents* [On-line]. Available: www.alz.org

American Psychiatric Association. (1994). *Diagnostic and statistical manual of mental disorders* (4th ed.). Washington, DC: American Psychiatric Press.

Beck, C., Heacock, P., Mercer, S.O., Walls, R.C., Rapp, C.G., & Vogelpohl, R.S. (1997). Improving dressing behavior in cognitively impaired nursing home residents. *Nursing Research, 46,* 126–132.

Benjamin, B.J. (1999). Validation: A communication alternative. In L. Volicer & L. Bloom-Charette (Eds.), *Enhancing the quality of life in advanced dementia* (pp. 107–125). Philadelphia: Brunner/Mazel.

Bohling, H.R. (1991). Communication with Alzheimer's patients: An analysis of caregiver listening patterns. *International Journal of Aging and Human Development, 33,* 249–267.

Burgener, S.C. (1998). Quality of life in late-stage dementia. In L. Volicer & A. Hurley (Eds.), *Hospice care for patients with advanced progressive dementia* (pp. 88–113). New York: Springer.

Burgener, S.C., Jirovec, M., Murrell, L., & Barton, D. (1992). Caregiver and environmental variables related to difficult behaviors in institutionalized, demented elderly persons. *Journal of Gerontology, 47,* P242–P249.

Fiatarone, M.A., O'Neill, E.F., Doyle, N., Clements, K.M., Roberts, S.B., Kehayias, J.J., Lipsitz, L.A., & Evans, W.J. (1993). The Boston FICSIT study: The effects of resistance training and nutritional supplementation on physical frailty in the oldest old. *Journal of the American Geriatrics Society, 41,* 333–337.

Folstein, M.F., Folstein, S.E., & McHugh, P.R. (1975). "Mini-mental state": A practical method for grading the cognitive state of patients for the clinician. *Journal of Psychiatric Research, 12,* 189–198.

Franssen, E.H., Kluger, A., Torossian, C.L., & Reisberg, B. (1993). The neurologic syndrome of severe Alzheimer's disease: Relationship to functional decline. *Archives of Neurology, 50,* 1029–1039.

Gerdner, L.A., Hall, G.R., & Buckwalter, K.C. (1996). Caregiver training for people with Alzheimer's based on a stress threshold model. *Image: The Journal of Nursing Scholarship, 28,* 241–246.

Greiner, F., English, S., Dean, K., Olson, K.A., Winn, P., & Beatty, W.W. (1997). Expression of game-related and generic knowledge by dementia patients who retain skill at playing dominoes. *Neurology, 49,* 518–523.

Hall, G.R., & Buckwalter, K.C. (1987). Progressively lowered stress threshold: A conceptual model for care of adults with Alzheimer's disease. *Archives of Psychiatric Nursing, 1,* 399–406.

Jones, J.M., & Jones, K.D. (1997). Promoting physical activity in the senior years. *Journal of Gerontological Nursing, 23*(7), 40–48.

Klein, A., & Kowall, N. (1998). Alzheimer's disease and other progressive dementias. In L. Volicer & A. Hurley (Eds.), *Hospice care for patients with advanced progressive dementia* (pp. 3–28). New York: Springer.

Kovach, C.R., & Henschel, H. (1996). Planning activities for patients with dementia: A descriptive study of therapeutic activities on special care units. *Journal of Gerontological Nursing, 22*(9), 33–38.

Lawton, M.P. (1982). Competence, environmental press, and the adaptation of older people. In M.P. Lawton, P.G. Windley, & T.O. Byerts (Eds.), *Aging and the environment: Theoretical approaches* (pp. 33–59). New York: Springer.

Lawton, M.P. (1995). Quality of life in Alzheimer's disease. *Alzheimer's Disease and Associated Disorders, 8*(Suppl. 3), 138–150.

Leidy, N.K. (1994). Functional status and the forward progress of merry-go-rounds: Toward a coherent analytical framework. *Nursing Research, 43,* 196–202.

Logsdon, R.G., & Teri, L. (1997). The Pleasant Events Schedule-AD: Psychometric properties and relationship to depression and cognition in Alzheimer's disease patients. *Gerontologist, 37,* 40–45.

Morris, J.N., Mahoney, E.K., Murphy, K., Gornstein, E.S., Ruchlin, H.S., & Lipsitz, L. (1998). A randomized controlled nursing intervention to maintain functional status in nursing home residents. *Canadian Journal of Quality in Health Care, 14*(3), 14–22.

Omnibus Budget Reconciliation Act of 1987, PL 101-203, 42 C.F.R. § 483.25 *et seq.*

Potatacke, R. (1993). *Nanny's special gift.* New York: Paulist Press.

Quayhagen, M.P., Quayhagen, M., Corbeil, R.R., Roth, P., & Rodgers, J.A. (1995). A dyadic remediation program for care recipients with dementia. *Nursing Research, 44,* 153–159.

Rader, J. (1995). Balancing the benefit and burden of interventions. In J. Rader & E.M. Tornquist (Eds.), *Individualized dementia care* (pp. 95–100). New York: Springer.

Raia, P. (1999). Habilitation therapy: A new starscape. In L. Volicer & L. Bloom-Charette (Eds.), *Enhancing the quality of life in advanced dementia* (pp. 21–37). Philadelphia: Brunner/Mazel.

Sacks, O. (1985). *The man who mistook his wife for a hat and other clinical tales.* New York: Summit Books.

Silverio, E., & Koenig-Coste, J. (1999). "Let's talk about it": Early stage concerns. Paper presented at Quality of Life for Persons with Dementia meeting, Bedford, MA, March 31, 1999.

Souren, L.E., Franssen, E.H., & Reisberg, B. (1997). Neuromotor changes in Alzheimer's disease: Implications for patient care. *Journal of Geriatric Psychiatry and Neurology, 10*(3), 93–98.

Stehman, J.M., Strachan, G.I., Glenner, J.A., Glenner, G.G., & Neubauer, J.K. (1996). *Handbook of dementia care*. Baltimore: The Johns Hopkins University Press.

Stone, J., Wyman, J.F., & Salisbury, S.A. (1999). *Clinical gerontological nursing: A guide to advanced practice* (2nd ed.). Philadelphia: W.B. Saunders.

Tideiksaar, R. (1998). *Falls in older persons: Prevention & management* (2nd ed., pp. 68–70). Baltimore: Health Professions Press.

Trudeau, S.A. (1999). Prevention of physical impairment in persons with advanced Alzheimer's disease. In L. Volicer & L. Bloom-Charette (Eds.), *Enhancing the quality of life in advanced dementia* (pp. 80–90). Philadelphia: Brunner/Mazel.

Volicer, L., Hurley, A.C., & Camberg, L. (1999). A model of psychological well-being in advanced dementia. *Journal of Mental Health and Aging, 5*(1), 83–94.

Volicer, L., Hurley, A.C., Lathi, D.C., & Kowall, N.W. (1994). Measurement of severity in advanced Alzheimer's disease. *Journal of Gerontology, 49*, M223–M226.

Volicer, L., Hurley, A.C., & Mahoney, E. (1995). Management of behavioral symptoms of dementia. *Nursing Home Medicine, 12*(3), 300–306.

Volicer, L., Hurley, A.C., & Mahoney, E. (1998). Behavioral symptoms of dementia. In L. Volicer & A. Hurley (Eds.), *Hospice care for patients with advanced progressive dementia* (pp. 68–87). New York: Springer

Volicer, L., Seltzer, B., Rheaume, Y., Fabiszewski, K.J., Herz, L.R., Shapiro, R., & Innis, P. (1987). Progression of Alzheimer-type dementia in institutionalized patients: A cross-sectional study. *Journal of Applied Gerontology, 6*, 83–94.

Wahl, J. (1994). *I remember! cried Grandma Pinky*. Mahwah, NJ: Bridgewater Books.

# 3

# Mood Disorders

Mrs. Clark is an 80-year-old woman who has become less interested in her social activities and has stopped attending church services. She has become reclusive, has started to neglect her hygiene, and is losing weight. Her family and friends have become concerned, so her daughter, Cecilia, takes her to a physician. During the examination, Mrs. Clark knows her name, the date, and where she is, but is not able to remember any new information and is not able to explain proverbs, which indicates a deficit in abstract thinking. During the examination, Mrs. Clark complains of poor sleep, lack of appetite, and feeling tired. She says her life is not worth living and reports that she has considered taking "a pill to end it all." She does not have any psychiatric history. Mrs. Clark is diagnosed with depression and is prescribed an antidepressant.

## EPIDEMIOLOGY OF MOOD DISORDERS

Depression is quite common in the general population, affecting 2%–4% of individuals. It is even more common in individuals seen in a general medical practice (5%–10%) or hospitalized for medical reasons (10%–14%). Older adults are susceptible to depression because of personal losses and health problems. As many as 25% of elderly individuals report symptoms ranging from chronic mild unhappiness to full-blown depression. It is estimated that up to 40% of medically ill older adult nursing facility residents have undiagnosed depression (Depression Guideline Panel, 1993a).

Bipolar disorders are less common than depression, affecting 0.4%–1.2% of individuals. The age of onset usually is in the early 20s, but bipolar disorders can occur throughout the life span. There seems to be a strong genetic component that predisposes people to developing bipolar disorder (Depression Guideline Panel, 1993b). Mania or hypomania was reported to occur in 5%–10% of elderly patients referred for the treatment of affective disorder. Sixty percent of elderly patients who present with a manic episode have memory impairment, and the diagnosis of "cerebral organic impairment" is made in 24% of them (Young & Klerman, 1992).

An episode of depression in an older adult individual with no prior history of depression may indicate an insidious onset of dementia. Sometimes, however, severe depression may be mistaken for a dementing illness. Depression in dementia is quite common (Wragg & Jeste, 1989). Symptoms of depression include

- Depressed mood lasting longer than 2 weeks, which often is described as overwhelming sadness or emptiness
- An increase or a decrease in appetite or weight
- Sleeping too much or too little
- Feeling either agitated or slowed down
- Loss of interest in usual activities
- Lack of energy
- Feelings of worthlessness and guilt
- Difficulty thinking and concentrating
- Thoughts of death or suicide

Depression, which is a serious illness, leads to death by suicide in 15% of depressed individuals and increases the death rate from medical causes of residents in institutions (Rovner et al., 1991).

## TYPES OF MOOD DISORDERS

The two main types of mood disorders are depression and bipolar disorder. It is important to differentiate between these two conditions because antidepressant treatment in individuals with bipolar disorder may lead to manic episodes and rapid, cyclical changes between depression and mania.

### DEPRESSIVE DISORDERS

It is possible to differentiate several types of depression that differ in severity and symptoms (American Psychiatric Association, 1994). The types are major depressive disorder, dysthymic disorder, adjustment disorder with depressed mood, and depressive disorder not otherwise specified.

## Major Depressive Disorder

Major depressive disorder is an episode of persistent depression lasting at least 2 weeks. It involves depressed mood and loss of interest in usual activities as well as other symptoms of depression, most commonly decreased sleep and decreased appetite (Table 3.1). Major depressive disorder usually starts in adolescence or the mid-20s and may lead to several episodes of depression throughout the person's life.

There are several subgroups of major depressive disorder. Psychotic depression is a major depression combined with hallucinations or delusions. These delusions often are self-accusatory or paranoid. Treatment of psychotic depression often requires both antidepressants and antipsychotics. Seasonal affective disorder is characterized by episodes of depression that repeatedly occur at the same time of the year. It is more common during the winter and may be related to decreased light exposure. Seasonal affective disorder occurs mainly in women and may respond to bright light exposure and other forms of therapy. Atypical depression is a chronic mood disorder that involves increased sleep and increased appetite. It sometimes responds better to treatment with monoamine oxidase inhibitors than to treatment with other antidepressants.

## Dysthymic Disorder

Dysthymia is a disorder in which the symptoms of depression are less severe than in major depression but are more chronic and last for at least 2 years. Some individuals report that they believe that they were depressed their entire lives.

## Adjustment Disorder with Depressed Mood

Adjustment disorder with depressed mood is a pathological reaction to psychosocial stress or loss. The most common losses in elderly individuals are death of a spouse and loss of independence as a result of physical disability or institutionalization. Depressed mood in response to these losses is a normal reaction. If the depressed mood lasts more than 2 months and is accompanied by other symptoms of depression, then psychological therapy may be required.

## Depressive Disorder Not Otherwise Specified

The category of depressive disorder not otherwise specified encompasses disorders with depressive features that do not meet the criteria for the previ-

**Table 3.1.  Diagnostic criteria for major depressive episode and dysthymic disorder**

| Symptoms | Major depressive episode[a] | Dysthymic disorder[b] |
| --- | --- | --- |
| Depressed mood | Most of the day, nearly every day (by report or observation) | Most of the day, for more days than not |
| Diminished interest or pleasure | In all or almost all activities most of the day nearly every day | |
| Change in appetite | Nearly every day, or weight loss or weight gain when not dieting | Poor appetite or overeating |
| Sleep abnormality | Insomnia or hypersomnia nearly every day | Insomnia or hypersomnia |
| Psychomotor changes | Psychomotor agitation or retardation nearly every day, observable by others | |
| Fatigue | Fatigue or loss of energy nearly every day | Low energy or fatigue |
| Self-image disturbance | Feeling of worthlessness or excessive or inappropriate guilt nearly every day | Low self-esteem |
| Cognitive disturbance | Diminished ability to think or concentrate, or indecisiveness, nearly every day | Poor concentration or difficulty making decisions |
| Despair | Recurrent thoughts of death, recurrent suicidal ideation with or without plan, or suicide attempt | Feelings of hopelessness |

[a]Five or more of the listed symptoms (at least one of them must be 1 or 2) during the same 2-week period representing a change from previous functioning.

[b]Symptom 1 and two or more additional symptoms for at least 2 years.

ously mentioned disorders and that have specific diagnostic criteria. Depressive disorders not otherwise specified include premenstrual dysphoric disorder; minor depressive disorder; recurrent brief depressive disorder; postpsychotic depressive disorder of schizophrenia, a major depressive episode superimposed on delusional disorder or schizophrenia; and situations in which the clinician has concluded that a depressive disorder is present but is unable to determine whether it is primary, caused by a general medical condition, or substance induced.

Two depressive disorders that are particularly relevant for older adults are minor depressive disorder and recurrent brief depressive disorder. Minor depressive disorder is characterized by depressive episodes of at least 2 weeks but with fewer than the five items that are required for a diagnosis of major depressive disorder. An episode involves either a sad or depressed mood or loss of interest or pleasure in nearly all activities and a total of two to four symptoms that characterize major depressive disorder. The symptoms must cause clinically significant distress or impairment in social, occupational, or other important areas of functioning.

Recurrent brief depressive disorder consists of depressive episodes lasting from 2 days to 2 weeks, occurring at least once a month for 12 months. The diagnostic criteria are the same as those for major depressive disorder except for duration of symptoms. The periods of depressed mood must cause significant distress or impairment in social, occupational, or other important areas of functioning.

## BIPOLAR DISORDER

Bipolar disorder is a condition in which depressive episodes alternate with manic episodes. Manic episodes are distinct periods of persistently elevated, abnormally expansive, or irritable mood associated with at least three of the following symptoms: inflated self-esteem/grandiosity, markedly decreased need for sleep, increased talkativeness (pressured speech), flight of ideas (rapidly racing thoughts), marked distractibility, increased goal-directed activity/psychomotor agitation, and excessive involvement in pleasurable activities without regard for negative consequences (e.g., buying sprees, sexual indiscretions). Symptoms must be severe enough to seriously impair function or to require hospitalization to prevent harm to self and others (Depression Guideline Panel, 1993b). If all of the symptoms are present but they are not severe enough to impair function or warrant hospitalization, then the diagnosis is "hypomanic episode."

Four types of bipolar disorders are recognized in the *Diagnostic and Statistical Manual of Mental Disorders, Fourth Edition* (DSM-IV; American Psychiatric Association, 1994): bipolar I disorder, bipolar II disorder, cyclothymic disorder, and bipolar disorder not otherwise specified. Bipolar II disorder differs from bipolar I disorder by the exhibition of only hypomanic episodes rather than manic ones. Cyclothymic disorder is characterized by numerous hypomanic episodes alternating with depressive symptoms that are of insufficient number, severity, or pervasiveness of duration to meet criteria for a major depressive episode. Bipolar disorder not otherwise specified includes rapid alteration of manic and depressive symptoms, hypomanic episodes without intercurrent depressive symptoms, and situations in which the bipolar disorder results from a general medical condition or is substance induced.

## TREATMENT OF MOOD DISORDERS

Three treatment modalities for depression are available: antidepressant medications, psychotherapy, and electroconvulsive therapy. Treatment with antidepressants is indicated in people with moderate to severe major depressive disorder. Psychotherapy alone is recommended for treatment of people with mild to moderate major depression. Combination therapy of antidepressants and psychotherapy may be required in people with partial responses to either treatment alone and for those with a chronic history of depression and poor interepisode recovery. Electroconvulsive therapy is a first-line treatment option only for people with severe or psychotic forms of major depression, those who fail to respond to other therapies, those who have medical conditions precluding the use of medications, and those with a need for rapid response (Depression Guideline Panel, 1993b). Mood stabilizers are drugs of choice for the treatment of bipolar disorders.

### ANTIDEPRESSANTS

Several types of antidepressants are available (Table 3.2), and other antidepressants are being developed. The choice of medication is based on side effect profiles, history of prior response, family history of response, type of depression, concurrent medical or psychiatric illnesses, and currently prescribed medications. It is always important to start with a low dose and gradually increase it. Most antidepressants do not exert their full effect until 2–3 weeks after initiation of the treatment, but some people have reported an almost immediate effect, if not relief, from depressive symptoms.

### Tricyclic Antidepressants (Tricyclics)

Tricyclics are the oldest form of antidepressant medication. In addition to their antidepressant effect, they often produce undesirable side effects because they affect chemicals (neurotransmitters) that brain cells use to communicate with one another. Tricyclics block the effect of acetylcholine, and this action may cause dryness of the mouth, constipation, and difficulties in urination that sometimes escalate to urinary retention. Because acetylcholine is an important component for memory (see Chapter 1), tricyclics may aggravate memory deficit in people with mild dementia. Other undesirable effects include postural hypotension and abnormal cardiac rhythms, an especially dangerous effect in people who are taking antiarrhythmic medications. Because of these undesirable effects, tricyclics are used less frequently as the drugs of first choice. They are much less expensive, however, than newer agents. Amitriptyline (Elavil, Endep) and nortriptyline (Aventyl, Pamelor) are preferable to other tricyclics because they have fewer side effects. Doxepin (Adapin, Sinequan) has a sedating effect in addition to its antidepressant

### Table 3.2.  Antidepressant medications

| Drug class[a] | Name (trade name) | Dose range (mg) | Frequency[b] | Elimination half-lives (hours) |
|---|---|---|---|---|
| Tricyclics | Amitriptyline (Elavil, Endep) | 25–100 | TID | 24 |
| | Doxepin (Adapin, Sinequan) | 25–100 | TID, HS (up to 150 mg) | 17 |
| | Nortriptyline (Aventyl, Pamelor) | 25–50 | BID–QID | 26 |
| MAOIs | Phenelzine (Nardil) | 15–30 | TID | 2 |
| | Tranylcypromine (Parnate) | 10–20 | BID–TID | 2 |
| SSRIs | Fluoxetine (Prozac) | 10–40 | QAM | 168 |
| | Fluvoxamine (Luvox) | 50–300 | QHS | 15 |
| | Paroxetine (Paxil) | 20–50 | QAM/HS | 24 |
| | Sertraline (Zoloft) | 50–200 | QAM/HS | 24 |
| Other | Mirtazapine (Remeron) | 15–45 | QHS | 30 |
| | Nefazodone (Serzone) | 50–300 | BID | 3 |
| | Trazodone (Desyrel) | 50–600 | TID, HS (up to 300 mg) | 8 |
| | Venlafaxine (Effexor) | 25–75 | BID–TID | 11 |

[a] MAOIs, monoamine oxidase inhibitors; SSRIs, selective serotonin reuptake inhibitors.

[b] QD, once a day; BID, twice a day; TID, three times a day; QID, four times a day; QAM, every morning; QHS, every evening.

effect, and the sedation may be useful in people who have difficulties in sleeping (see Chapter 11).

## Monoamine Oxidase Inhibitors

Monoamine oxidase inhibitors (MAOIs) act by inhibiting the breakdown of some neurotransmitters involved in depression, especially serotonin and norepinephrine. MAOIs are recommended if the person does not respond to, or does not tolerate, other antidepressants; if there is a family or personal history of positive response to MAOIs; and if the depression has atypical symptom features (e.g., increased appetite, increased sleep). Administration of MAOIs requires adherence to a strict diet because MAOIs in combination with certain cheeses and other foods containing tyramine may dangerously increase blood pressure. People taking MAOIs must avoid certain medications, such as cold and cough medicines containing vasoconstrictors and decongestants, meperidine, and possibly other narcotic drugs.

## Selective Serotonin Reuptake Inhibitors

Serotonin is a neurotransmitter that plays an important role in mood, appetite, and sleep. Lack of serotonin may lead to the development of depressive disorders. Inhibition of serotonin reuptake increases its effect on nerve cells and improves mood. Selective serotonin reuptake inhibitors (SSRIs) are safe and well tolerated. The most common side effects of SSRIs are stomach upset and diarrhea. There are four SSRIs: fluoxetine (Prozac), fluvoxamine (Luvox), paroxetine (Paxil), and sertraline (Zoloft). All of them are equally effective, although there are some individual differences in patient responses. Sertraline may be the first drug of choice because it is the least likely to cause side effects. Fluoxetine has a long half-life and its administration sometimes causes agitation and anxiety, and paroxetine increases the effects of some other medications by inhibiting their breakdown in the liver. Inhibition of medication breakdown may lead to toxic reaction or an increased incidence of side effects.

## Other Antidepressants

This group includes heterocyclics, with a chemical structure different from tricyclics. Heterocyclics include trazodone (Desyrel) and nefazodone (Serzone), which inhibit the uptake of both serotonin and norepinephrine, another neurotransmitter involved in the regulation of mood. Trazodone is less effective for the treatment of depression than are the other antidepressants, but it has a strong sedative effect that may be beneficial for people with difficulties in sleeping. Nefazodone does not have this sedative effect but may also normalize the sleep pattern.

Another antidepressant is venlafaxine (Effexor), which also inhibits the uptake of both serotonin and norepinephrine and does not have as many gastrointestinal side effects as SSRIs. Venlafaxine, however, may cause a sustained increase in blood pressure that may be undesirable in a person with hypertension. Mirtazapine (Remeron) is an antidepressant that increases the release of both serotonin and norepinephrine by nerve cells. Studies indicate that mirtazapine is as effective as other antidepressants (Kasper, 1995). Its most common side effects are sedation, increased appetite, weight gain, constipation, and dizziness.

## PSYCHOTHERAPY

Psychotherapy is effective as an antidepressant therapy in people with mild to moderate major depressive episodes (Depression Guideline Panel, 1993b). The effectiveness of psychotherapy, however, may be decreased in people with mild to moderate dementia. Psychotherapy is not indicated for people with melancholic features (e.g., loss of interest or pleasure, psychomotor disturbances, worse depression in the morning, early morning awakening). The psychotherapeutic course should be time limited and involve at least once-a-week visits. If there is no improvement in 6 weeks or only partial improvement in

12 weeks, then a consultation with a psychiatrist for initiation of pharmacological therapy may be required.

Psychotherapy may involve a variety of verbal and nonverbal techniques and procedures that may have different objectives. Although there are more than 250 types of psychotherapy, only cognitive therapy, behavior therapy, interpersonal therapy, and brief dynamic therapy have been rigorously evaluated. The combination of psychotherapy and antidepressant treatment is more effective than either treatment alone.

### Cognitive Therapy

The goal of cognitive therapy is to alleviate the symptoms of depression by identifying and correcting a person's negative thought patterns and to prevent relapse by correcting personal beliefs or schemas. A meta-analysis of studies comparing cognitive therapy in depressed outpatients with drug treatment and placebo showed that cognitive therapy was effective in 50% of patients and was more effective than no therapy or the administration of a placebo (Depression Guideline Panel, 1993b). It is not clear whether individual cognitive therapy is more effective than group cognitive therapy.

### Behavior Therapy

Behavior therapy is based on a functional analysis of behavior, social learning theory, or both. The strategies include activity scheduling, self-control therapy, social skills training, and problem solving. The overall efficacy of behavior therapy was found to be 55% and was similar in individual and group settings (Depression Guideline Panel, 1993b).

### Interpersonal Psychotherapy

The goal of interpersonal psychotherapy is to clarify and resolve one or more interpersonal difficulties, such as role dispute, social isolation, prolonged grief reaction, or role transition. Interpersonal difficulties are understood to cause and/or maintain depression. Initially, education about the nature and course of depression also is provided to the patient or client. One study found interpersonal psychotherapy to be more effective than placebo or cognitive therapy (Elkin et al., 1998).

### Brief Dynamic Psychotherapy

Brief dynamic psychotherapy is not designed specifically for depression. Instead, it aims to resolve depressive symptoms by resolving core conflicts based on the patient's or client's personality and situational variables. A meta-analysis of six trials indicates that the overall efficacy of brief dynamic psychotherapy is 35% and that it may be less effective than other psychotherapeutic strategies.

## ELECTROCONVULSIVE THERAPY

Electroconvulsive therapy (ECT) is indicated in the treatment of severe depression with intense prolonged symptoms, severe vegetative symptoms, marked functional impairment, and psychotic symptoms. ECT is indicated if several adequate trials of medication are unsuccessful. Approximately 50%–70% of individuals who do not respond to medication typically will respond to ECT. ECT may be especially effective in people with melancholic features. People who have been treated successfully with ECT should receive maintenance antidepressant therapy because without such treatment, 30%–60% will experience another depressive episode.

## MOOD STABILIZERS

Lithium and some anticonvulsants are used to treat bipolar disorder (Table 3.3). The anticonvulsants that are used in people with dementia include valproic acid, carbamazepine, and gabapentin. No information is available about the use of lamotrigine and topiramate, both of which have mood-stabilizing properties, in individuals with dementia who are experiencing a manic or hypomanic episode.

### Lithium

Lithium (e.g., Eskalith, Lithobid) is a drug of choice for the treatment of bipolar disorders in young individuals. The use of lithium in older individuals is questionable because they may have age-related reduced lithium clearance, decreased kidney function, or diseases and drug treatments that affect lithium excretion. Other disorders also may predispose older adults to lithium toxicity, even with plasma levels below 1.5 mEq/liter. The adverse effects of lithium include fine hand tremor, polyuria, and thirst. Transient and mild nausea also are observed. Some evidence exists that lithium is less effective in older adults with "organic manic disorder," dementia, or mania complicated by serious medical conditions or by other psychiatric diagnoses (Young, 1997).

### Valproic Acid

Valproic acid (Depakene), or its better tolerated enteric-coated derivative, divalproex sodium (Depakote), is used widely in the treatment of bipolar disorders in young individuals. It can be used alone or in combination with lithium. The potential side effects of valproic acid include sedation, weight gain, hair loss, thrombocytopenia, and hepatic dysfunction. A study of geriatric nursing facility patients with dementia, bipolar affective disorder, or both concluded that treatment with valproic acid produces better results with fewer side effects than treatment with lithium (Conney & Kaston, 1999). In addi-

**Table 3.3.   Mood stabilizers**

| Name (trade name) | Dose range (mg) | Frequency[a] | Elimination half-life (hours) | Therapeutic level |
|---|---|---|---|---|
| Lithium (Eskalith, Lithobid, and others) | 100–300 | BID–QID | 22 | 0.6–1.2 mEq/l |
| Valproic acid (Depakene); divalproex sodium (Depakote) | 100–300 | BID–QID | 9–16 | 50–125 μg/ml |
| Carbamazepine (Tegretol) | 100–200 | BID | 25–65 (12–17)[b] | 4–12 μg/ml |
| Gabapentin (Neurontin) | 300–600 | TID[c] | 5–7 | Not measured |

[a] BID, twice a day; TID, three times a day; QID, four times a day.

[b] After chronic administration.

[c] After titration phase (during titration, 300 mg once a day or BID).

tion, treatment with lithium is more expensive than treatment with valproic acid because of the need to carefully monitor plasma drug levels and side effects.

## Carbamazepine

Carbamazepine (Tegretol) also is used for treatment of bipolar disorders, although it may not be as effective as lithium and valproic acid. Carbamazepine may have fewer neurotoxic effects than lithium, but it has other adverse effects, including rash, sedation, ataxia, agranulocytosis, hepatic dysfunction, and electrolyte disturbance. Carbamazepine is effective in the treatment of agitation in nursing facility residents with dementia (Tariot, 1999).

## Gabapentin

Although support from the results of well-controlled trials is lacking, gabapentin (Neurontin) is used increasingly to treat bipolar disorders and in the management of behavior problems in people with dementia (Letterman & Markowitz, 1999). The advantages of gabapentin over other anticonvulsants are the relative lack of adverse effects with gabapentin and there is no need to monitor plasma drug levels. Gabapentin is used alone or in combination with neuroleptics.

Mrs. Clark started taking desipramine because it is less expensive than other antidepressants. When she complained of dry mouth, constipation, and sedation, Mrs. Clark's physician changed her medication to sertraline, which does not cause these problems. Mrs. Clark's mood improved, and she began to attend church again. Her memory and ability to cope with problems also improved, although there is a mild, persistent deficit. This deficit gradually worsened, however, even while normal mood and antidepressant use were maintained. A year later, Mrs. Clark was not able to handle money during grocery shopping, and she got lost on the way to church. A follow-up evaluation found evidence of moderate cognitive impairment, and she was referred to a neurologist. The reversible causes of dementia were excluded, and Mrs. Clark was diagnosed as having probable Alzheimer's disease.

# RELATIONSHIP BETWEEN MOOD DISORDERS AND DEMENTIA

## DEPRESSION AND DEMENTIA

The relationship between depression and dementia is quite complex. A history of depression early in life increases the risk for development of a progressive dementia in old age. Individuals with primary degenerative dementia who also are depressed are more likely to have relatives with a history of depression than are people with degenerative dementia who are not depressed. This indicates that there may be a common genetic mechanism for depression and primary degenerative dementia. Some studies indicate that apolipoprotein E heterogeneity may be the common factor, but there is no general agreement yet.

Depression and dementia are best seen as intersecting continua (Emery & Oxman, 1992). On one side is a "pure" depression that has no or only mild cognitive impairment. The other extreme is primary dementia with no affective changes. In most cases there is a combination of both conditions, and it may be difficult to distinguish which process is more important. The similarity between depression and dementia also is demonstrated by biochemical changes in the brain that indicate that similar neurotransmitters are affected in both conditions.

Several combinations of depression and dementia are possible. Five prototypical groups have been proposed (Emery & Oxman, 1992): major depression without depressive dementia, depressive dementia, degenerative dementia without depression, depression of degenerative dementia, and independent co-occurrence of degenerative dementia and depression.

## Major Depression Without Depressive Dementia

Mild cognitive impairment that is detectable by neuropsychological testing is quite common in people with major depressive disorder and may be explained by loss of interest and inability to concentrate on the task at hand, which are common symptoms of depression.

## Depressive Dementia

Some individuals develop symptoms of depression before any cognitive deficits are detected, but they also have a pronounced cognitive and functional impairment during a depressive episode. Treating depression leads to improvement in the cognitive and functional impairment together with lessening of the depression. This condition is sometimes labeled "pseudodementia of depression" and is considered one of the reversible types of dementia. Long-term follow-up, however, indicates that individuals with this reversible dementia have a 50% probability of developing a progressive dementia 3 years later and a 90% probability 10 years later. Depressive symptoms are common in people who eventually develop progressive dementia. In one study 72% of patients with an autopsy-confirmed diagnosis of Alzheimer's disease had experienced depression, changes in mood, social withdrawal, and suicidal ideation more than 2 years before the diagnosis of dementia was made (Jost & Grossberg, 1996).

## Degenerative Dementia Without Depression

Some people develop dementia with no changes in their mood and personality. This course may be more common in individuals who develop dementia late in life and who live in a sheltered environment that does not challenge their ability to act independently. These individuals commonly are unaware of their deficits.

## Depression of Degenerative Dementia

Symptoms of depression may develop in a person with progressive dementia without a previous diagnosis of depression. Making a diagnosis of depression in an individual with dementia is very difficult. Several symptoms of major depressive disorder (e.g., diminished interest, change in appetite, sleep abnormality, cognitive disturbance) are commonly seen during some stages of a progressive dementia. The detection of other symptoms (e.g., fatigue, self-image disturbance, despair) relies on self-report, which is not possible in individuals with language or comprehension impairments. As a result, reports of the incidence of depression in individuals with dementia vary widely, ranging from 15% to 57%. The diagnosis of depression in a person with dementia can be made by observing the person's expression, obtaining information about emotional lability exhibited by periods of tearfulness or crying, and evaluating eating and sleeping patterns. The symptoms of depression may differ according to gender. Men tend to exhibit more apathy and vegetative signs, whereas women show more reclusiveness and emotional lability (Ott, Tate, Gordon, & Heindel, 1996).

## Independent Co-occurrence of Degenerative Dementia and Depression

Because both depression and dementia are common conditions, it is possible that they occur in the same individual by chance alone. The prevalence of depression, however, decreases with age. For example, the Epidemiologic Catchment Area study found major depression in only 1% of individuals 65 years old or older (Kessler, Cleary, & Burke, 1999). In contrast, the prevalence of dementia increases with age from 5%–10% in individuals older than age 65 to 47% in individuals older than age 85. In agreement with these data, the prevalence ratio of dementia to depression in nursing facility residents is as much as 10 to 1. These data indicate that even though it is possible that dementia and depression are unrelated, in most older adult individuals with depression there may be an underlying dementing process.

## MANIC AND HYPOMANIC EPISODES

The prevalence of manic episodes in people with Alzheimer's disease is relatively low, and most of the individuals with manic episodes had a history of mania before the onset of Alzheimer's disease (Lyketsos, Corazzini, & Steele, 1995). Manic episodes are more common in people with cerebrovascular disease, especially when it involves the right hemisphere and orbitofrontal cortex (Shulman & Herrmann, 1999). The manic symptoms in people with Alzheimer's disease are related to their unawareness of behavior problems that is independent of the severity of the dementia (Starkstein, Sabe, Chemerinski, Jason, & Leiguarda, 1996). Mood enhancers are drugs of choice in the treatment of these symptoms.

> Two years after her diagnosis, Mrs. Clark was admitted to a hospital after she was found on the floor, unconscious. She was found to have a urinary tract infection and to be dehydrated. She recovered and was discharged home. Her antidepressant was stopped because she no longer complained of being sad. Mrs. Clark's family feels that giving her antidepressants is not necessary and is just a waste of money. Her daughter, Cecilia, however, observed that Mrs. Clark cries occasionally for no apparent reason. Within a few weeks, Mrs. Clark was unable to sleep

during the night and was refusing food. She also experienced periods of restlessness during which she called out, "Help me! Help me!" Mrs. Clark is angry with Cecilia and her other caregivers, and she sometimes tries to hit them.

## CONSEQUENCES OF DEPRESSION IN ADVANCED DEMENTIA

The treatment of depression in individuals with dementia requires the long-term administration of antidepressants. The antidepressant treatment may compensate for neurochemical changes induced by dementia, and because these changes are progressive, there is a high probability of recurrent depression if the treatment is ceased. This also is true in Alzheimer's disease and other progressive dementias. As the dementia progresses, individuals may be increasingly less able to express their feelings of depression verbally. There are, however, two main areas in which continuing depression expresses itself—vegetative symptoms and behavioral consequences.

Vegetative symptoms include food refusal and sleep abnormality. The management of vegetative symptoms is described in more detail in Chapters 10 and 11. Behavioral consequences include restlessness, agitation, repetitive vocalization, irritability, and combative behavior. Irritable mood in children and adolescents is accepted by DSM-IV as an equivalent of depressed mood. The progression of primary dementias, such as Alzheimer's disease, can be viewed as the reverse of human development because abilities and skills learned early in life are retained longer than are skills learned later. People with dementia lose the most complex functional abilities early in the disease process and the more basic skills later. It is possible that this reverse development also leads to equivalence of irritable and depressed moods. Irritability leads to decreased tolerance for environmental stimuli and may be one of the reasons for resistive and combative behavior (see Chapters 9 and 12). "Anger attacks," which were inhibited by antidepressant treatment, were described in middle-age individuals (Fava et al., 1993) and may be the underlying mechanism for catastrophic reactions that occur in some individuals with dementia.

Antidepressants are effective in the treatment of depression even in individuals with advanced dementia. An open study showed that sertraline improved both mood and food intake in individuals with severe dementia (Volicer, Rheaume, & Cyr, 1994). Antidepressants that produce sedation as a side effect (e.g., trazodone) are useful in the treatment of insomnia in individuals with dementia who also are depressed. Trazodone also was found to decrease irritability, anxiety, restlessness, and affective disturbance when administered three times a day (Lebert, Pasquier, & Petit, 1994).

Because of crying spells and other symptoms, Mrs. Clark was restarted on her antidepressant. This treatment gradually improved her mood and sleep. It also decreased her restlessness, food refusal, and assaultive behavior.

## REFERENCES

American Psychiatric Association. (1994). *Diagnostic and statistical manual of mental disorders* (4th ed.). Washington, DC: American Psychiatric Press.

Conney, J., & Kaston, B. (1999). Pharmacoeconomic and health outcome comparison of lithium and divalproex in a VA geriatric nursing home population: Influence of drug-related morbidity on total cost of treatment. *American Journal of Managed Care, 5*(2), 197–204.

Depression Guideline Panel. (1993a). *Depression in primary care: Detection and diagnosis.* Rockville, MD: Agency for Health Care Policy and Research.

Depression Guideline Panel. (1993b). *Depression in primary care: Treatment of major depression.* Rockville, MD: Agency for Health Care Policy and Research.

Elkin, I., Shea, T.M., Watkins, J.T., Imber, S.D., Sotsky, S.M., Collins, J.F., Glass, D.R., Pilkonis, P.A., Leber, W.R., Docherty, J.P., Fiester, S.J., & Parloff, M.B. (1998). National Institute of Mental Health Treatment of Depression Collaborative Research Program: General effectiveness of treatments. *Archives of General Psychiatry, 46,* 971–982.

Emery, V.O., & Oxman, T.E. (1992). Update on the dementia spectrum of depression. *American Journal of Psychiatry, 149,* 305–317.

Fava, M., Rosenbaum, J.F., Pava, J.A., McCarthy, M.K., Steingard, R.J., & Bouffides, E. (1993). Anger attacks in unipolar depression. I: Clinical correlates and response to fluoxetine treatment. *American Journal of Psychiatry, 150,* 1158–1163.

Jost, B.C., & Grossberg, G.T. (1996). The evolution of psychiatric symptoms in Alzheimer's disease: A natural history study. *Journal of the American Geriatrics Society, 44,* 1078–1081.

Kasper, S. (1995). Clinical efficacy of mirtazapine: A review of meta-analyses of pooled data. *International Clinical Psychopharmacology, 10*(Suppl. 4), 25–35.

Kessler, L.G., Cleary, P.D., & Burke, J.D. (1999). Psychiatric disorders in primary care. *Archives of General Psychiatry, 42,* 583–587.

Lebert, F., Pasquier, F., & Petit, H. (1994). Behavioral effects of trazodone in Alzheimer's disease. *Journal of Clinical Psychiatry, 55,* 536–538.

Letterman, L., & Markowitz, J.S. (1999). Gabapentin: A review of published experience in the treatment of bipolar disorder and other psychiatric conditions. *Pharmacotherapy, 19,* 565–572.

Lyketsos, C.G., Corazzini, K., & Steele, C. (1995). Mania in Alzheimer's disease. *Journal of Neuropsychiatry and Clinical Neuroscience, 7,* 350–352.

Ott, B.R., Tate, C.A., Gordon, N.M., & Heindel, W.C. (1996). Gender differences in the behavioral manifestations of Alzheimer's disease. *Journal of the American Geriatrics Society, 44,* 583–587.

Rovner, B.W., German, P.S., Brant, L.J., Clark, R., Burton, L., & Folstein, M.F. (1991). Depression and mortality in nursing homes. *Journal of the American Medical Association, 265,* 993–996.

Shulman, K.I., & Herrmann, N. (1999). Bipolar disorder in old age. *Canadian Family Physician, 45,* 1229–1237.

Starkstein, S.E., Sabe, L., Chemerinski, E., Jason, L., & Leiguarda, R. (1996). Two domains of anosognosia in Alzheimer's disease. *Journal of Neurology, Neurosurgery and Psychiatry, 61,* 485–490.

Tariot, P.N. (1999). Treatment of agitation in dementia. *Journal of Clinical Psychiatry, 60*(Suppl. 8), 11–20.

Volicer, L., Rheaume, Y., & Cyr, D. (1994). Treatment of depression in advanced Alzheimer's disease using sertraline. *Journal of Geriatric Psychiatry and Neurology, 7,* 227–229.

Wragg, R.E., & Jeste, D.V. (1989). Overview of depression and psychosis in Alzheimer's disease. *American Journal of Psychiatry, 146,* 577–587.

Young, R.C. (1997). Bipolar mood disorders in the elderly. *Psychiatric Clinics of North America, 20,* 121–136.

Young, R.C., & Klerman, G.L. (1992). Mania in late life: Focus on age at onset. *American Journal of Psychiatry, 149,* 867–876.

# 4

# Delusions and Hallucinations

Mr. Dimple, a 65-year old former postal worker, retired a year ago because of memory problems. He stays home alone because his wife, Donna, still works. Several months ago, he began to accuse Donna of having an affair. He also complained that the neighbors were stealing his tools from the garage. Donna explained to her husband that she was not having an affair because she spent all of her time either working or being with him. She also pointed out that his tools are in the basement work-shop—that he probably took them there and simply forgot about them. Mr. Dimple, however, persisted in his accusations. Donna persuaded her husband that he needed a routine physical examination. She explained her husband's groundless accusations to Dr. Doherty, the primary provider. Dr. Doherty examined Mr. Dimple and found him to be gener-ally physically healthy. He then tested Mr. Dimple's cognitive ability and found short-term memory deficit, impaired judgment, and decreased spatial orientation. Dr. Doherty referred Mr. Dimple for neurological evaluation. The evaluation ruled out reversible causes of dementia, and a diagnosis of probable Alzheimer's disease was made.

Mr. Dimple experiences paranoid delusions. *Delusion* is a false belief, based on incorrect inference about an external reality, that is firmly sustained despite what almost everyone believes and despite evidence that constitutes incontrovertible and obvious proof to the contrary (American Psychiatric Association, 1994). Delusions often are combined with hallucinations. *Hallucinations* are sensory perceptions occurring without the appropriate stimulation of the corresponding sensory organ. Paranoid delusions are common psychotic symptoms in Alzheimer's disease. Paranoid delusions and auditory hallucinations were present in the 51-year-old woman first described by Dr. Alois Alzheimer in 1906. A study of 228 patients with Alzheimer's disease reported that 52% showed evidence of delusions or hallucinations (Hirono et al., 1998). Most of them had only delusions (80%), some had both delusions and hallucinations (18%), and few had only hallucinations (2%). Delusions and hallucinations, however, also may be caused by other conditions.

## CONDITIONS THAT CAUSE
## DELUSIONS AND HALLUCINATIONS

The most common causes of delusions and hallucinations in younger individuals are schizophrenia and psychotic depression, but the most common cause in older individuals is dementia. A retrospective review of patients 65 years old and older who were admitted to a geriatric psychiatry service, however, indicated that multiple other problems can cause delusions and hallucinations (Webster & Grossberg, 1999). Dementia was present in 40% of these patients. The second most common cause of psychotic symptoms was major depression, diagnosed by chart review in 33% of the subjects. It is possible, however, that some of the patients diagnosed as depressed also have dementia because depression is very common in individuals with mild dementia (see Chapter 3).

Another common cause of delusions and hallucinations (Webster & Grossberg, 1999) is delirium (7% of study subjects) that is induced either by medical conditions (e.g., urinary tract infection, cellulitis) or by drugs (e.g., anticholinergic agents, benzodiazepines, alcohol). Other medical conditions that can cause delusions and hallucinations are electrolyte imbalance, hyperglycemia, seizure disorder, hypothyroidism, and Parkinson's disease. Other causes of delusions and hallucinations are bipolar disorder (5%), drug toxicity (4%), delusional disorder (2%), schizophrenia (1%), and schizoaffective disorder (1%).

It is especially important to rule out drugs as a cause of delusions and hallucinations. Many classes of drugs can cause psychotic symptoms in older people, most commonly antiparkinsonian drugs, anticholinergic and antihistaminic agents, tricyclic antidepressants, and stimulants. Benzodiazepines and alcohol may cause psychotic symptoms, not only by their acute effects but also as symptoms of their withdrawal. Other classes of drugs that may produce psychotic symptoms include anticonvulsants, steroids, antiarrhythmics, and drugs used for the treatment of peptic ulcer disease.

## EPIDEMIOLOGY OF DELUSIONS AND HALLUCINATIONS

Delusions and hallucinations occur at all stages of Alzheimer's disease, and, when present in the early stages of the disease, they may precipitate diagnostic evaluation (Jost & Grossberg, 1996). Estimates of delusion prevalence in Alzheimer's disease vary widely, ranging from 10% to 73% in different studies (Leuchter & Spar, 1985). This variation results from different diagnostic criteria for dementia and delusions and from different study populations.

Delusions may be divided into two types—simple persecutory delusions and complex, bizarre, or multiple delusions (Burns, Jacoby, & Levy, 1990). Simple persecutory delusions include those of theft or suspicion. Suspicions involve beliefs such as being watched or having an unfaithful spouse. Complex delusions may include the conviction that a family member or pet is injured, that plots against individuals of a certain religious faith are being made, or that wild parties are happening on a nonexistent floor of the nursing facility. An example of a complex delusion is Capgras syndrome, which consists of a false belief that significant people have been replaced by identical impostors. Complex delusions also may present as grandiose delusions that often are connected with euphoria and hypomanic mood.

The most common delusions in people with Alzheimer's disease are paranoid delusions, and the most common of those, occurring in about 28% of cases, are delusions of theft (Rubin, 1992). The cause of delusions may be attributable to a person's memory deficit because he or she, for example, may have forgotten where personal belongings were placed. Delusions of suspicion are observed in 9% of people with Alzheimer's disease, and more complex delusions are observed in 3.6%. A common delusion of suspicion is that other residents in a long-term care facility are criticizing the individual behind his or her back. A stimulus for this delusion may be an innocent conversation in the hallway that is not heard very well by the resident, who subsequently misinterprets it. Another common delusion is the belief that the person is much younger than his or her actual age. This delusion may be connected with misidentification. For example, a man may think that his wife is his mother. Delusions are more common in men than in women, in African Americans than in Caucasians, in individuals with impaired hearing, and in individuals with a low level of education (Rao & Lyketsos, 1998).

Hallucinations occur in 25%–30% of people with Alzheimer's disease and are even more common in people with dementia with Lewy bodies (Ala, Yang, Sung, & Frey, 1997), in whom hallucinations often are presenting symptoms and are among the diagnostic indicators. Onset of hallucinations in

Alzheimer's disease usually occurs later in the disease progression, typically more than 5 years after the onset of dementia (Hope, Keene, Fairburn, Jacoby, & McShane, 1999) or more than 1 year after diagnosis (Jost & Grossberg, 1996). In approximately half of the individuals, hallucinations are temporary, but in others, hallucinations persist until death (Hope et al., 1999). It is important, therefore, to frequently reevaluate the need for pharmacological treatment in individuals with dementia. Hallucinations and delusions are associated with greater functional impairment, and they are more common in individuals who have extrapyramidal signs such as muscle rigidity or myoclonus (Jost & Grossberg, 1996).

## ETIOLOGY OF DELUSIONS AND HALLUCINATIONS

Four reasons are proposed for the occurrence of delusions and hallucinations in individuals with dementia (Berrios, 1989):

1.  An intercurrent confusional state (delirium)
2.  An interaction of dementia and personality
3.  A separate mental disorder that coexists with the dementia
4.  A disinhibition of cortical functions resulting in "released" symptomatology

It is important to eliminate the first reason because the confusional state could be caused by a reversible medical condition, such as drug toxicity or electrolyte imbalance. The interaction between dementia and personality is covered in Chapter 1 and is an important factor in the clinical management of individuals with dementia. Some individuals who develop Alzheimer's disease and other progressive dementias have histories of psychiatric disorders that precede any cognitive impairment. Such a disorder (e.g., schizophrenia) may recur during the course of dementia and lead to pronounced delusions and hallucinations. In most individuals, however, delusions and hallucinations are a consequence of the damage done to brain cortical areas by dementia.

Delusions probably are related to limbic system damage, especially damage to the caudate nucleus and temporal lobes of the brain (Cummings, 1992). The limbic system regulates arousal and participates in monitoring the environment. Limbic system dysfunction interferes with assessment of the environment, and incorrect assessment of danger may result. This misinterpretation of the environment may be manifested as paranoid behavior resulting in persecutory ideation and inappropriate fear. Limbic system participation in generating delusions and hallucinations is supported by the greater density of senile plaques and neurofibrillary tangles in the limbic structures of patients who have delusions and hallucinations (Zubenko et al.,

1991). Patients with delusions also have more extensive calcification of basal ganglia, more abnormal electroencephalograms, and lower cerebral blood flow in the temporal lobes than do patients without delusions (Rao & Lyketsos, 1998).

The limbic system is innervated by neurons in brain stem nuclei that use either dopamine or acetylcholine for communication with other brain cells. A disturbed balance between dopamine and acetylcholine input may be the cause of delusions and hallucinations. Delusions and hallucinations occur when dopamine input is increased or acetylcholine input is decreased or both. Increased dopamine input occurs when people with Parkinson's disease are treated with levodopa (e.g., Sinemet). The purpose of levodopa administration in this condition is to replace dopamine deficiency. In some individuals, however, levodopa treatment leads to the development of hallucinations because dopamine levels become temporarily too high.

Alzheimer's disease also affects the balance between dopamine and acetylcholine input, but in a different way than Parkinson's disease. Alzheimer's disease primarily damages the brain stem nuclei that use acetylcholine, causing acetylcholine deficiency and a relative preponderance of dopamine. The role of dopamine in the development of delusions and hallucinations also is supported by the finding that patients with a specific genetic variation of dopamine receptor were more at risk for developing delusions and hallucinations than patients who had a different genetic variation of this receptor (Sweet et al., 1998).

As expected, delusions and hallucinations in Alzheimer's disease are improved by drugs that either inhibit dopamine effects or enhance acetylcholine effects. Drugs that inhibit dopamine effects (neuroleptics) are the drugs that are used most often to treat delusions and hallucinations. They are discussed later in this chapter. Acetylcholine effects can be enhanced by inhibiting the acetylcholine breakdown that is mediated by the enzyme cholinesterase. Cholinesterase inhibitors are approved for the treatment of Alzheimer's disease because of their effect on cognitive functioning. One of these inhibitors, metrifonate, also significantly decreases hallucinations in patients with Alzheimer's disease (Cummings, 1997). With the relentless progression of Alzheimer's disease, however, cholinesterase inhibitors ultimately lose their effectiveness.

Mr. Dimple was started on 0.5 mg of risperidone once a day and his delusions resolved. His dementia, however, progressed, and he now requires assistance with the activities of daily living. He also lost the ability to recognize members of his family. Mr. Dimple looks for his wife when she is present and accuses her of being an impostor. He does not cooperate when she provides care for him, and he becomes verbally aggressive toward her.

## RELATIONSHIP OF DELUSIONS AND HALLUCINATIONS TO OTHER BEHAVIORAL SYMPTOMS OF DEMENTIA

Several investigators have studied the relationship between delusions and hallucinations and other behavioral symptoms of dementia. In general, two types of behavior are related to delusions and hallucinations, and the relationship may differ according to the gender of the individual with dementia.

Several studies reported that aggression is related to the occurrence of delusions and hallucinations (Haupt, Janner, Ebeling, Stierstorfer, & Kretschmar, 1998; Kunik et al., 1999), although one study found that physical aggression is predicted by sad facial affect (McShane, Keene, Fairburn, Jacoby, & Hope, 1998). In McShane et al.'s study, persecutory ideas predicted motor hyperactivity. A relationship between agitation and paranoid delusions also has been reported, but only in men (Cohen et al., 1993). Another study reported that agitation is related to misidentification, such as phantom-boarder syndrome, Capgras-like syndrome, and "one's house is not one's home" misidentification (Haupt et al., 1998).

The discrepancies in these reports probably are the result of different definitions of aggression and agitation. Some investigators consider all behavioral symptoms of dementia to be "agitation" (Cohen-Mansfield, Marx, & Rosenthal, 1989). Further discussion of the differences between aggression and agitation and why resistiveness is a more appropriate concept than aggression is included in Chapters 9 and 12. In any case, overwhelming clinical evidence indicates that delusions and hallucinations are significant causes of other behavior problems in individuals with dementia.

> Donna reported her problems in providing care for her husband to Dr. Doherty. The physician recommended that Donna join a support group for caregivers of people with Alzheimer's disease, which was organized by the local chapter of the Alzheimer's Association. Donna attends weekly meetings and has learned that her problems are not unique. She also has learned strategies that other caregivers use to decrease problem behaviors during care. For example, she learned not to insist on providing care when her husband refused it and to come back later when he may be more willing to cooperate.

## TREATMENT OF DELUSIONS AND HALLUCINATIONS

Although potent and effective medications for treatment of delusions and hallucinations are available, it is best to avoid using them unless they are determined to be absolutely necessary. It is important to identify the presence of delusions and hallucinations and their importance relative to other behavioral symptoms. Some individuals with dementia have many delusions and vivid hallucinations but are neither bothered by them nor negatively affected by them behaviorally. An example of such a delusion is misidentification of one's reflection in a mirror as another person. Although some people may be bothered by mirrors and become upset, others talk to or vocalize at their reflection, and this encounter becomes a meaningful activity. This activity may be especially meaningful for gay or lesbian individuals, who may consider their reflection to be a lover.

If delusions and hallucinations are identified as a cause of other behavior problems, then pharmacological treatment is necessary. The first step to take, however, should be controlling the consequences of delusions and hallucinations using nonpharmacological approaches (Volicer, Mahoney, & Brown, 1998).

## NONPHARMACOLOGICAL APPROACHES

In a consensus paper on the management of agitation, which included aggression, nonpharmacological approaches were divided into three categories (Nasr & Osterweil, 1999):

1.  Sensory interventions by staff that affect people's senses (e.g., hearing aids that may decrease auditory delusions)
2.  Environmental modification or redesign that changes either the physical or social environment. Physical modifications include adequate lighting, decreased noise, and avoidance of restraints; social modifications include providing safe space for ambulation and forming homogeneous resident populations. The behaviors that are caused by delusions and hallucinations are more easily tolerated on a special care dementia unit than in a general nursing facility environment because these behaviors often are distressing for residents who are cognitively intact.
3.  Behavior strategies using operant conditioning or cognitive techniques. Operant conditioning may use differential reinforcement, antecedent modification, or positive reinforcement strategies; cognitive techniques may use reminiscence/life review and validation therapy.

The most important component of any nonpharmacological approach is careful attention to proper communication strategies. An appropriate approach to communication may significantly decrease the impact of delusions and hallucinations. The principles of successful communication include the following (Raia, 1999):

1.  Recognizing that behavior cannot be changed by words because the person cannot understand reasoning and does not remember what he or she

was told—The only way to change a person's behavior is to change the caregiver's behavior or the environment.

2. Avoiding the use of the word "no"—Instead of arguing with the older adult with dementia, it is better to attempt change or to modify the person's behavior by distracting him or her.

3. Avoiding reality orientation and accepting the person's reality—For instance, it is better to empathize with an individual who complains that something was stolen from her than to try to persuade her that she just misplaced the object.

4. Always making the person as comfortable as possible—This includes smiling and using a positive tone of voice, saying something positive about the person (e.g., commenting on clothing), acknowledging the person's emotions, and answering in a positive way, even though the person's speech does not make sense.

Another approach to the management of behaviors uses the RESPECT model (Maxfield, Lewis, & Cannon, 1996). The components of this model for caregiver education are Recognize, Empathize, Support, Prevent, Enhance, Care, and Take time.

Donna was able to manage her husband's behavior problems for some time; however, eventually, he refused to be bathed at all and when she tried to help him wash, he threatened to hit her. This became a particular problem because Mr. Dimple was occasionally incontinent of urine. Dr. Doherty increased the risperidone dose. This increased dosage made Mr. Dimple more likely to permit care, but he became more rigid and walked with a shuffling gait. Dr. Doherty stopped the risperidone and started him on olanzapine. Mr. Dimple's muscle rigidity and shuffling gait improved, but olanzapine was less effective in controlling his resistiveness during care. At one point, Mr. Dimple pushed Donna, and she fell and broke her arm. As a consequence, Mr. Dimple was admitted to a nursing facility, where he is cared for by two caregivers at a time. Sometimes he requires lorazepam to decrease his anxiety. He believes that he is working at the post office and spends most of the day carrying around newspapers and magazines—delivering mail. With the progression of his dementia, his resistiveness gradually decreased; olanzapine was tapered off and eventually stopped.

## PHARMACOTHERAPEUTIC APPROACHES

The medications that are used most commonly in treating delusions and hallucinations are neuroleptic agents. The older neuroleptics act by blocking dopamine receptors in the brain. Dopamine is a neurotransmitter that is prominently involved in generating delusions and hallucinations. The older neuroleptics are called "typical" because they act in a similar manner and differ from one another mainly in their side effect profiles. The newer neuroleptics, called "atypical," have less effect on dopamine receptors than typical neuroleptics, but they also affect other neurotransmitters, such as serotonin, histamine, and norepinephrine. Representative drugs from each category are listed in Table 4.1.

### Typical Neuroleptics

A large number of medications belong to the class of typical neuroleptics, but they have a high incidence of adverse reactions that limit their long-term use. The most common typical neuroleptic used is haloperidol (Haldol). An advantage of haloperidol is that it is relatively fast acting and is available for parenteral administration. Haloperidol, however, has a high incidence of extrapyramidal side effects, such as muscle rigidity, shuffling gait, and blunt affect. It also commonly causes tardive dyskinesia (Jeste, Rockwell, Harris, Lohr, & Lacro, 1999), a condition that is characterized by involuntary movement of the mouth, tongue, and other parts of the body. Tardive dyskinesia is a disabling and disfiguring condition that interferes with functioning, especially the ability to eat and swallow. An alternative to haloperidol, if intramuscular administration is necessary, is loxapine (Loxitane), which is chemically different from other typical neuroleptics and may have some atypical neuroleptic characteristics (Carlyle, Ancill, & Sheldon, 1993).

Thioridazine (Mellaril) does not produce extrapyramidal side effects, but it may cause dry mouth and urinary retention because it blocks acetylcholine

**Table 4.1. *Selected drugs used in treating delusions and hallucinations***

| Drug class | Name (trade name) | Dose range (mg) | Frequency[a] | Elimination half-life (hours) |
|---|---|---|---|---|
| Typical neuroleptics | Haloperidol (Haldol) | 0.5–1 | QD–TID | 18 |
| | Thioridazine (Mellaril) | 10–40 | QD–TID | 4 |
| | Loxapine (Loxitane) | 5–10 | BID–TID | 4 |
| Atypical neuroleptics | Risperidone (Risperdal) | 0.25–1 | QD–BID | 3–20 (21–30)[b] |
| | Olanzapine (Zyprexa) | 2.5–10 | QD | 30 |
| | Quetiapine (Seroquel) | 25–100 | BID–TID | 6 |
| Benzodiazepines | Lorazepam (Ativan) | 0.5–1 | QD–TID | 14 |
| | Oxazepam (Serax) | 10–20 | QD–TID | 7 |

[a]QD, once a day; BID, twice a day; TID, three times a day.
[b]active metabolite.

receptors. Thioridazine also produces postural hypotension, cardiac arrhythmias, and sedation. The sedative effect may be beneficial in agitated individuals. All typical neuroleptics are equally effective in the treatment of behaviors that are related to delusions and hallucinations in Alzheimer's disease (Helms, 1985), but they are, for the most part, being replaced by atypical neuroleptics.

## Atypical Neuroleptics

Atypical neuroleptics are becoming the drugs of choice in treating delusions and hallucinations. These drugs have fewer side effects and only rarely do they lead to tardive dyskinesia (Jeste et al., 1999). In individuals with schizophrenia atypical neuroleptics are effective against the positive symptoms of the disease (hallucinations), and they improve the negative symptoms, which include apathy, affective flattening, and social withdrawal. This improvement in negative symptoms also may be significant for people with Alzheimer's disease who develop similar negative symptoms.

The available atypical neuroleptics are clozapine (Clozaril), risperidone (Risperdal), olanzapine (Zyprexa), and quetiapine (Seroquel). Additional atypical neuroleptics are being developed. Clozapine is the oldest atypical neuroleptic and is a drug that may cause the least number of extrapyramidal side effects. It is rarely used, however, because it may produce agranulocytosis and requires frequent blood tests. Risperidone is similar to haloperidol except that it does not cause extrapyramidal side effects when given in low doses (up to 1 mg/day), which usually are sufficient to control delusions and hallucinations in people with Alzheimer's disease (Katz et al., 1999). Risperidone is converted into an equally potent metabolite; however, the rate of metabolism is highly variable because some individuals have very low cytochrome $P_{450}IID_6$ activity as a result of genetic polymorphism. Some people develop extrapyramidal side effects with higher doses, and they may experience postural hypotension. Even with these possible side effects, risperidone is becoming the drug of choice in the treatment of delusions and hallucinations in individuals with dementia.

Olanzapine has a sedating effect and may block acetylcholine receptors. It is less likely to produce extrapyramidal side effects than risperidone, but it may still produce them in people with dementia with Lewy bodies (Walker et al., 1999). Olanzapine is effective in improving behavioral symptoms of dementia in nursing facility populations, but the lowest dose (5 mg) used in one study was more effective than were higher doses (Grossberg et al., 1999). Olanzapine is long acting; therefore, it takes several days to build up an effective drug concentration. A loading dose regimen, however, is sometimes used in people with acute schizophrenia if rapid onset of olanzapine action is required. This regimen uses a dose that is four times higher than the maintenance dose on Day 1, three times higher on Day 2, and two times higher on

Day 3, and a regular dose on Day 4 and beyond. It is not clear whether such an approach is suitable for people with dementia, who benefit most from a low dose.

Quetiapine is the most recent atypical agent as of this writing, and there is little experience with its use in individuals with dementia. A single uncontrolled trial in men and women who were at least 65 years old and who had a psychotic disorder found that psychotic symptoms improved with doses of quetiapine ranging from 25 to 800 mg/day (McManus, Arvanitis, & Kowalcyk, 1999). The most common side effects are somnolence, dizziness, postural hypotension, and agitation. Extrapyramidal side effects occur in 6% of individuals taking queitapine. A possible disadvantage of quetiapine is the need for ophthalmological examinations, which is suggested by the development of cataracts in dogs (Stip & Boisjoly, 1999).

## Other Drugs

The management of an episode of resistiveness to care or a catastrophic reaction that is elicited by delusions or hallucinations sometimes requires short-term antianxiety therapy. This therapy is needed especially during the initial period after neuroleptics are initiated and before the titration period is completed. Short-acting benzodiazepines, such as lorazepam (Ativan) or oxazepam (Serax), are preferable to long-acting benzodiazepines, such as diazepam (Valium), because long-acting benzodiazepines tend to accumulate and cause sedation and lethargy in older individuals. Another class of drugs that may be useful in decreasing the behavior problems induced by delusions and hallucinations are mood stabilizers (see Chapter 3).

## REFERENCES

Ala, T.A., Yang, K.H., Sung, J.H., & Frey, W.H., II. (1997). Hallucinations and signs of parkinsonism help distinguish patients with dementia and cortical Lewy bodies from patients with Alzheimer's disease at presentation: A clinicopathological study. *Journal of Neurology, Neurosurgery and Psychiatry, 62,* 16–21.

American Psychiatric Association. (1994). *Diagnostic and statistical manual of mental disorders* (4th ed.). Washington, DC: American Psychiatric Press.

Berrios, G. (1989). Non-cognitive symptoms in the diagnosis of dementia: Historical and clinical aspects. *British Journal of Psychiatry, 154*(Suppl. 4), 11–16.

Burns, A., Jacoby, R., & Levy, R. (1990). Psychiatric phenomena in Alzheimer's disease. II: Disorders of perception. *British Journal of Psychiatry, 157,* 76–81.

Carlyle, W., Ancill, R.J., & Sheldon, L. (1993). Aggression in the demented patient: A double-blind study of loxapine versus haloperidol. *International Clinical Psychopharmacology, 8*(2), 103–108.

Cohen, D., Eisdorfer, C., Gorelick, P., Luchins, D., Freels, S., Semla, T., Paveza, G., Shaw, H., & Ashford, J.W. (1993). Sex differences in the psychiatric manifestations of Alzheimer's disease. *Journal of the American Geriatrics Society, 41,* 229–232.

Cohen-Mansfield, J., Marx, M.S., & Rosenthal, A.S. (1989). A description of agitation in a nursing home. *Journal of Gerontology: Medical Sciences, 44,* M77–M84.

Cummings, J. (1992). Psychosis in neurologic disease, neurobiology and pathogenesis. *Neuropsychiatry, Neuropsychology, and Behavioral Neurology, 5,* 144–150.

Cummings, J.L. (1997). Changes in neuropsychiatric symptoms as outcome measures in clinical trials with cholinergic therapies for Alzheimer disease. *Alzheimer Disease and Associated Disorders, 11,* S1–S9.

Grossberg, G., Jackson, J., Tariot, P., Fraser, M., Jacobs, L., Carroll, R., Smith, D., Sherman, D., Torgerson, D., & Siegal, A. (1999). Managing elderly patients with acute behavioral changes in the long-term care setting. *Annals of Long-Term Care, 7*(Suppl. 5), 1–10.

Haupt, M., Janner, M., Ebeling, S., Stierstorfer, A., & Kretschmar, C. (1998). Presentation and stability of noncognitive symptom patterns in patients with Alzheimer disease. *Alzheimer Disease and Associated Disorders, 2,* 323–329.

Helms, P.M. (1985). Efficacy of antipsychotics in the treatment of the behavioral complications of dementia: Review of the literature. *Journal of the American Geriatrics Society, 33,* 206–209.

Hirono, N., Mori, E., Yasuda, M., Ikejiri, Y., Imamura, T., Shimomura, T., Ikeda, M., Hashimoto, M., & Yamashita, H. (1998). Factors associated with psychotic symptoms in Alzheimer's disease. *Journal of Neurology, Neurosurgery and Psychiatry, 64,* 648–652.

Hope, T., Keene, J., Fairburn, C.G., Jacoby, R., & McShane, R. (1999). Natural history of behavioural changes and psychiatric symptoms in Alzheimer's disease—a longitudinal study. *British Journal of Psychiatry, 174,* 39–44.

Jeste, D.V., Rockwell, E., Harris, M.J., Lohr, J.B., & Lacro, J. (1999). Conventional vs. newer antipsychotics in elderly patients. *American Journal of Geriatric Psychiatry, 7,* 70–76.

Jost, B.C., & Grossberg, G.T. (1996). The evolution of psychiatric symptoms in Alzheimer's disease: A natural history study. *Journal of the American Geriatrics Society, 44,* 1078–1081.

Katz, I.R., Jeste, D.V., Mintzer, J.E., Clyde, C., Napolitano, J., & Brecher, M. (1999). Comparison of risperidone and placebo for psychosis and behavioral disturbances associated with dementia: A randomized, double-blind trial. *Journal of Clinical Psychiatry, 60,* 107–115.

Kunik, M.E., Snow-Turek, A.L., Iqbal, N., Molinari, V.A., Orengo, C.A., Workman, R.H., & Yudofsky, S.C. (1999). Contribution of psychosis and depression to behavioral disturbances in geropsychiatric inpatients with dementia. *Journals of Gerontology, Series A: Biological Sciences and Medical Sciences, 54,* M157–M161.

Leuchter, A.F., & Spar, J.E. (1985). The late onset psychoses. *Journal of Nervous and Mental Disease, 173,* 488–494.

Maxfield, M.C., Lewis, R.E., & Cannon, S. (1996). Training staff to prevent aggressive behavior of cognitively impaired elderly patients during bathing and grooming. *Journal of Gerontological Nursing, 22*(1), 37–43.

McManus, D.Q., Arvanitis, L.A., & Kowalcyk, B.B. (1999). Quetiapine, a novel antipsychotic: Experience in elderly patients with psychotic disorders. *Journal of Clinical Psychiatry, 60,* 292–298.

McShane, R., Keene, J., Fairburn, C., Jacoby, R., & Hope, T. (1998). Psychiatric symptoms in patients with dementia predict later development of behavioural abnormalities. *Psychological Medicine, 28,* 1119–1127.

Nasr, S.Z., & Osterweil, D. (1999). The nonpharmacologic management of agitation in the nursing home: A consensus approach. *Annals of Long-Term Care, 7*(5), 171–180.

Raia, P. (1999). Habilitation therapy: A new starscape. In L. Volicer & L. Bloom-Charette (Eds.), *Enhancing the quality of life in advanced dementia* (pp. 21–37). Philadelphia: Brunner/Mazel.

Rao, V., & Lyketsos, C.G. (1998). Delusions in Alzheimer's disease: A review. *Journal of Neuropsychiatry, 10,* 373–382.

Rubin, E.H. (1992). Delusions as part of Alzheimer's disease. *Neuropsychiatry, Neuropsychology and Behavioral Neurology, 5,* 108–113.

Stip, E., & Boisjoly, H. (1999). Quetiapine: Are we overreacting in our concern about cataracts (the beagle effect)? *Canadian Journal of Psychiatry, 44*(5), 503.

Sweet, R.A., Nimgaonkar, V.L., Kamboh, I., Lopez, O.L., Zhang, F., & DeKosky, S.T. (1998). Dopamine receptor genetic variation, psychosis, and aggression in Alzheimer disease. *Archives of Neurology, 55,* 1335–1340.

Volicer, L., Mahoney, E., & Brown, E.J. (1998). Nonpharmacological approaches to the management of the behavioral consequences of advanced dementia. In M. Kaplan & S.B. Hoffman (Eds.), *Behaviors in dementia: Best practices for successful management* (pp. 155–176). Baltimore: Health Professions Press.

Walker, Z., Grace, J., Overshot, R., Satarasinghe, S., Swan, A., Katona, C.L., & McKeith, I.G. (1999). Olanzapine in dementia with Lewy bodies: A clinical study. *International Journal of Geriatric Psychiatry, 14,* 459–466.

Webster, J., & Grossberg, G.T. (1999). Late-life onset of psychotic symptoms. *American Journal of Geriatric Psychiatry, 6,* 196–202.

Zubenko, G.S., Moossy, J., Martinez, A.J., Rao, G., Claassen, D., Rosen, J., & Kopp, U. (1991). Neuropathologic and neurochemical correlates of psychosis in primary dementia. *Archives of Neurology, 48,* 619–624.

# 5

# Dependence in Activities of Daily Living

Activities of daily living (ADLs) are the activities that are needed for self-care and independent living. They include instrumental activities of daily living (IADLs) and physical activities of daily living (PADLs). Knowledge about factors that affect ADL function in people with dementia and about caregiving strategies that promote function is growing, although a gap still exists between that knowledge and clinical practice. This chapter provides guidelines for strengthening the link between dynamic assessment and clinical decisions because they guide how care is given.

Dementia is a progressive disease in which both cognitive and physical decline are hallmarks. Nevertheless, not all ADL dependence is attributable to dementia. Performance of ADLs can be facilitated by applying available knowledge; even a temporary improvement in independence increases the quality of life for people with dementia and their caregivers (Beck et al., 1997; National Citizens Coalition for Nursing Home Reform, 1986). People's ability to perform ADLs influences their quality of life and need for services. A focus on function allows caregivers to be supportive and to prevent unnecessary dependence. For people with dementia who live in the community, functional status is an important determinant of their ability to remain at home and their need for services. Nursing facilities, under the Nursing Home Reform

Act (Subtitle C of the Omnibus Budget Reconciliation Act of 1987), must provide care that assists each resident in attaining and maintaining his or her maximum practical functional status (Morris et al., 1998). This mandate requires proactive ADL–enhancing care.

> Eugenia Ewing is a 78-year-old woman who lives in the city on the fifth floor of an apartment building for older adults. There is an elevator two doors down the hall from her apartment, and a bus line runs on her street. She loves the one-bedroom apartment where she has lived for 13 years. The apartment is small but ample. She has it fixed up just the way she likes it, full of family pictures, plants, and remembrances from her large family and many friends. She knows all of her neighbors, and every Saturday afternoon there is music downstairs in the function room. Twice a week, a community-sponsored van takes the residents shopping, and the driver even helps carry bags of groceries. Friends visit every afternoon. They drink iced tea and share stories. In the evening, she usually eats a light supper and watches the news and a television show or two before going to bed.

## ASSESSMENT

A good assessment provides a guide for clinical decision making. Assessment of functional status tracks changes over time and assists in setting realistic goals by describing remediable functional deficits (Stone, Wyman, & Salisbury, 1999). Assessment includes the nature of the self-care deficit, the factors that contribute to it, and the person's remaining self-care abilities. A variety of scales to assess functional status in community and institutional settings exist (Gallo, Reichel, & Andersen, 1995; Morris et al., 1990; Morris, Fries, et al., 1997), and several excellent reviews have been published (Beck & Frank, 1997; Morris, Nonemaker, et al., 1997; Spector, 1997). As mentioned previously, this chapter focuses on the relationship between assessment of functional status and clinical decision making. Therefore, rather than providing an exhaustive review, selected examples of assessments that generate useful information for planning and providing care to people with dementia who have a self-care deficit are included.

One important contribution (Leidy, 1994) identifies four dimensions of functional status:

1. *Functional capacity*—the maximum potential to perform activities
2. *Functional performance*—the activities actually performed
3. *Functional reserve*—the difference between functional capacity and functional performance

4. *Functional capacity utilization*—the extent to which individuals are able to realize their potential

It has been observed (Beck & Frank, 1997) by applying this model to dementia that capacity and performance may not be equal in all situations. This raises interesting questions about what might account for capacity and performance differences, and whether caregiving interventions can bring performance up to the level of capacity.

## INSTRUMENTAL ACTIVITIES OF DAILY LIVING

IADLs are activities that are needed to support independent living. They include shopping, preparing meals, traveling, doing housework and laundry, using the telephone, taking medication, and managing money (Gallo et al., 1995; Lawton & Brody, 1969). IADLs are more complex and demand more cognitive skill than do basic ADLs. Therefore, they are impaired earlier in the progression of a dementia. At the same time, IADLs are meaningful in the everyday lives of all people, and it is important that people with dementia continue to participate in them to some extent for as long as possible (Stehman, Strachan, Glenner, Glenner, & Neubauer, 1996).

> Mr. Eaton, the building superintendent, stops by Mrs. Ewing's apartment to ask why she has not paid last month's rent. In reply, she gives Mr. Eaton $10.00 and thanks him for visiting. Although she is unsure who he is, she invites him in for tea and puts tap water and a tea bag in a cup for him. Mr. Eaton notices that Mrs. Ewing's plants are limp, as if overwatered. He asks her why her wet wash is hung over chairs all around the apartment. She replies that the dryer in the building is broken. (Mr. Eaton has not heard this report from any other resident.) Eunice, Mrs. Ewing's daughter, becomes upset when Mr. Eaton tells her of these events because every day, when she calls her mother, Eunice is assured by Mrs. Ewing that she is doing "just fine." Eunice makes an appointment for her mother at the Neighborhood Health Center (NHC).

Traditionally, assessment of IADLs has been made by self-report or proxy report, but the reliability of this approach has been questioned (Diehl, Marsiske, Horgas, & Saczynski, 1998; Karagiozis, 1998). (For a comprehensive discussion of these issues, see Beck & Frank, 1997, and Bennett, 1999.) An innovative and practical approach to assessment of IADLs is the Cognitive Performance Test (CPT) developed at the Minneapolis Veterans Administration Medical Center Geriatric Research, Education and Clinical Center (Burns, Mortimer, & Merchak, 1994). The CPT evaluates the degree to which particular deficits in information processing compromise common activities.

For example, the "toast test" evaluates the thinking and actions of a person who is asked to make toast. Six levels of function are described that form a continuum of how a person's thinking and functioning are related as he or she performs the test. Thus, the toast test helps to identify what the person can and cannot understand and do. The assessment can be performance based, by observing a person making toast, or informant based, by asking a caregiver to match the ability of the care recipient to a series of video vignettes depicting the six levels of function. The program is available on CD-ROM (Burns, Hepburn, Maddox, & Smith, 1998) and includes level-specific caregiving strategies that focus on the person's remaining abilities. Because the cognitive skills that are required to perform any task are similar (e.g., initiating, problem solving, sequencing, being aware of safety issues), the results of this assessment apply to many IADLs.

> A family meeting is organized at the NHC after Mrs. Ewing's evaluation. During the assessment, Mrs. Ewing is able to make toast without difficulty when the equipment is selected and set out for her. The NHC staff explain to Mrs. Ewing and Eunice that Mrs. Ewing still can safely perform concrete, familiar tasks and that it is important for Mrs. Ewing to continue to do as much as she is capable of doing independently. They begin to discuss the need for assistance with complex tasks that require planning, problem solving, or calculating. They also discuss the importance of continued monitoring and planning. Some existing resources are mobilized. For example, Eunice and her mother agree to pay the bills and do the laundry together, and a neighbor moves her daily visit to suppertime so she and Mrs. Ewing can make their shopping lists together. Other potential resources, such as Meals on Wheels and the local chapter of the Alzheimer's Association, are identified.

## PHYSICAL ACTIVITIES OF DAILY LIVING

Bathing, dressing, grooming, toileting, walking (mobility), and eating are the functional skills that are most often included in PADL scales. Most scales rate the level of dependence in each of these activities as a whole, although current knowledge shows that this is not sufficient for planning care. ADLs are complex. Each requires an individual to perform a number of discrete steps, often in a particular order, to complete the ADL successfully. Any individual step can be problematic, as can the sequencing of individual steps to complete the ADL. For example, 13 steps in handwashing (Tappen, 1994), 21 steps in toileting (Hutchinson, Leger-Krall, & Wilson, 1996), and 34 steps in dressing (Beck, 1988) have been identified.

PADL functional abilities decline in a predictable temporal order according to the complexity of the ADL—bathing, dressing, grooming, toileting, walking, and eating (Cohen-Mansfield, Werner, & Reisberg, 1995). Every person is unique and requires individualized assessment, but knowing this common pattern is useful in anticipatory problem solving and maximizing functional performance. For example,

- The most complex PADLs—bathing, dressing—need to be simplified first.
- People still may be able to eat with encouragement and verbal cues (no physical assistance) even if they require physical assistance with toileting.
- Ambulation can be maintained for a long time if risk factors for impaired mobility, such as deconditioning and medication side effects, are avoided.

People with dementia benefit from assessments that focus on the nature of self-care deficits that are unique to older adults. Most of the instruments that are commonly used to assess ADL function were developed within a physical disability perspective. They treat the ADL as a unitary, "all-or-none" activity, and rate people's degree of dependence on whether they require the assistance of others. This type of assessment is inadequate for people with dementia, for whom cognitive impairment is a more salient issue than physical impairment in performing ADLs, at least until they are well into the disease course. Furthermore, rating people as "dependent" provides inadequate information about the nature of their self-care deficit, no information about remaining self-care abilities, and no guidance about the kind of assistance that will promote functional performance. (See Beck and Frank, 1997, for a comprehensive discussion of this topic.) Two instruments are discussed in relation to these issues: the Minimum Data Set (MDS) and the Refined ADL Assessment Scale (RADL).

The MDS is mandated for use with all residents in nursing facilities that receive federal support. It includes ratings of ADL self-performance (independent, supervision, limited or extensive physical assistance) and level of physical support provided (none, setup, 1- or 2+-person physical assistance). When ADL performance requires any assistance, a more detailed assessment and care planning process that focuses on restorative care is triggered. Although this assessment is still conceptualized within a physical disability framework, and the category "supervision" includes three different methods of helping (oversight, encouragement, and cueing), the MDS and associated Resident Assessment Protocols (RAPS) represent a significant step toward the kind of assessment specificity that is necessary. The home care version (MDS-HC) (Morris, Fries, et al., 1997) is available for community-dwelling populations. It includes an assessment of informal support services that are available to the person being assessed. The MDS and MDS-HC are designed for use with all people receiving care.

Because people with dementia are a specialized group whose self-care performance is affected by the specific cognitive and physical impairments that are discussed in Chapter 2, we recommend a follow-up assessment of any self-performance deficit identified on the MDS using an instrument with enough specificity to guide care planning. For example, the RADL (Tappen, 1994) is designed specifically to assess both functioning and assistance required in five ADL tasks for people with dementia: toileting, washing, grooming, dressing, and eating. Each of these tasks is broken down into its component steps (ranging from 5 to 21), and the person's ability to perform each step is rated in terms of the five types of assistance that are needed to complete each step successfully: unassisted, verbal prompt, nonverbal prompt, physical guiding, or full assistance. Using the RADL, the caregiver is able to identify the particular component in which the person has difficulty and adjust the type and amount of assistance that are needed for the person to complete an ADL successfully (Tappen, 1994). ADL–specific functional performance measures also are available for dressing (Heacock, Beck, Souder, & Mercer, 1997) and eating (Tully, Matrakas, Muir, & Musallam, 1997).

## FACTORS AFFECTING ADL DEPENDENCE

Dementia is characterized by a progressive decline in cognitive and physical function (see Chapter 2). When these deficits are severe enough to interfere with daily activities, the person meets the diagnostic criteria for dementia that are listed in the *Diagnostic and Statistical Manual of Mental Disorders, Fourth Edition* (American Psychiatric Association, 1994). It is important to emphasize, however, that low cognitive test scores do not fully explain the level of ADL dependence observed in people with dementia (Beck et al., 1997). ADL performance occurs in the context of the interpersonal and physical environment, as depicted in the model of behavioral symptoms of dementia presented in the Introduction. These contextual factors can have positive or negative effects.

### CORE SYMPTOMS

Cognitive and physical impairments affect the person's ability to plan, initiate, maintain attention, sequence, solve problems, and complete the steps that are required for ADLs. IADLs are the first activities to be affected because of their heavy reliance on the executive functions of the brain.

The types of cognitive problems that affect dressing performance are deficits in perception, attention, initiation, memory, judgment, and apraxia (Beck, 1988). Different cognitive deficits yield a different type of problem with dressing. For example, the person with ideational apraxia may have difficulty in sequencing actions, whereas the person with ideomotor apraxia may know what to do but is unable to perform the motor movements or cannot respond to verbal instructions to carry out the necessary movements.

## Contextual Factors

A number of contextual factors affecting function are described in the literature. For example, the concept of "environmental press" has been described, which illustrates environmental influences on functioning (Lawton, 1983). Environmental influences increase as the person's functional status decreases, which is a stimulus for creating supportive environments. The positive contextual relationship between a caregiver's relaxed and smiling behavior and the older person's calm/functional behaviors during ADLs also is important (Burgener, Jirovec, Murrell, & Barton, 1992). Negative contextual attributes also have far-reaching negative effects on people with dementia. Common practices in facilities during mealtimes such as not providing the necessary assistance; creating a chaotic, high-stimulus environment; expectations of failure; using infantilizing behavior; and using ineffective feeding strategies provide dramatic testimony about the devastating consequences of the negative influence of context (Kayser-Jones, 1997; Kayser-Jones & Schell, 1997).

## Risk Factors for Functional Decline

Mrs. Ewing collapses in the hallway of her apartment building on a hot summer day, so her neighbors call 911. An ambulance takes her to the emergency room of the local hospital, where she is diagnosed with dehydration and delirium. She is admitted for intravenous therapy. Her care plan includes hydration, early mobilization, and avoidance of physical restraints. Her room is near the nurses' station. Motion sensors are placed under her mattress and seat cushion to alert staff when Mrs. Ewing gets up, so that assistance will be prompt. Her care plan includes balancing activity with rest, and she is encouraged to participate in ADLs to avoid excess disability and deconditioning.

Any acute change in function signals a medical problem. For example, sudden incontinence may be the result of a urinary tract infection or fecal impaction; a new difficulty in walking may reflect musculoskeletal, respiratory, or cardiovascular problems or weakness following an acute illness. Deconditioning occurs quickly with bed rest (see Chapter 2). A change in environment, including familiarity, structure, and routine, also is a risk factor for functional decline.

Even with the preventive care Mrs. Ewing receives in the hospital, her functional performance decreases, and she is no longer able to manage alone safely in her apartment. She is admitted to a nursing facility. Records from the NHC, interviews with Eunice, and direct assessment of Mrs. Ewing provide a more complete picture of her functional capacity and are used as a basis for care planning.

## INTERVENTIONS TO PROMOTE FUNCTIONAL PERFORMANCE

Supportive interventions improve the level of ADL performance in people with dementia (Beck et al., 1997; Morris et al., 1998). There is a growing body of knowledge about ways to maintain and improve ADL function in people with dementia. Several research programs provide specific guidelines for the care of people with dementia who have a particular self-care deficit. All of the interventions are based on three premises: 1) a philosophy of care that promotes dignity and prevents excess disability, 2) an emphasis on creating an environment that supports success, and 3) an understanding of cognitive and physical impairment effects on ADL functioning as a basis for targeting interventions to the underlying cause of the self-care deficit (see Chapter 2). Ongoing comprehensive assessment is necessary so that the care plan reflects the person's current functional ability and goals.

Time is a key issue for caregivers. Caregivers remark that more time is required when care recipients participate in their own care. Actually, the amount of increased time for many of these interventions is small. For example, clinically relevant improvement in dressing requires less than a 1-minute increase in nursing assistant time (Beck et al., 1997). Also, the time that is spent to maintain a person's current level of function is less than the amount of time it takes to care for the same person later, when that person's functional ability has decreased (Morris et al., 1998). Finally, current practice commonly allots too little time for some ADLs, which causes detrimental effects that could be avoided (Kayser-Jones, 1997; Morris et al., 1998). Federal regulations for nursing facilities clearly stipulate that quality of care includes "the necessary care and services to attain or maintain the highest practicable physical, mental, and psychosocial well-being" (Omnibus Budget Reconciliation Act of 1987, p. 395). A person's abilities in ADLs must be supported throughout the progression of a dementia. Approaches are needed that will encourage nursing facility administrators to adopt the use of independence-supporting strategies (Beck & Frank, 1997).

### SELECTED ADL-SPECIFIC INTERVENTIONS

Continued participation in IADLs is guided by issues of self-esteem, safety, and stress prevention. IADLs need to be greatly simplified, or the person may be able to participate in only some of the steps but not the entire activity (Stehman et al., 1996) (Table 5.1). Supportive services, such as a homemaker or Meals on Wheels, may allow a person who retains other instrumental skills to continue living in his or her own home (Stone et al., 1999). General principles of task simplifying, identifying the factors that affect ADL performance, and matching the assistance given to the assistance needed are important. For example

- Perform a comprehensive assessment, including specific self-care abilities and self-care deficits.
- Identify possible etiologies for limitations so that the interventions are directed to the cause whenever possible.
- Break down complex tasks into individual steps.
- Let the person complete one step before proceeding to the next step.
- Maintain a relaxed, unhurried pace.
- Create an environment that fosters success and pleasure.
- Give clear, simple directions (verbal or gestures), one at a time.
- Do not criticize the person.
- Smile and use positive feedback.

Remember that assistance comes in many forms: encouragement, verbal cues, visual cues (gestures), physical guidance (helping the person get started), and physical assistance. Match the type and amount of assistance to the person's level of performance of each step.

In the sections that follow, research that supports the functional performance of specific PADLs is highlighted. Strategies to maintain walking, such as exercise and the Merry Walker (Trudeau, 1999), are discussed in Chapter 2.

**Table 5.1.  Examples of IADL adaptations**

| IADL | Suggested adaptations |
|------|----------------------|
| Shopping | Plan and go shopping with others<br>Continue to help choose purchases |
| Meal preparation | Prepare one dish, with steps presented one at a time |
| Using the telephone | Help person list things to talk about before making a call<br>Help person call relatives and friends<br>Put pictures of people on preprogrammed telephone buttons |
| Money management | Simplify bill-paying routine<br>Carry small amounts of money<br>Make small purchases with assistance on shopping trips |

Adapted from Stehman, J.M., Strachan, G.I., Glenner, J.A., Glenner, G.G., & Neubauer, J.K. (1996). *Handbook of dementia care* (p. H IV: 14). Baltimore: The Johns Hopkins University Press.

## Bathing

Bathing is the most complex ADL, and therefore it is the first for which the person with dementia will require assistance. Interdisciplinary researchers are studying ways to make bathing less stressful for people with dementia and their caregivers (Sloane et al., 1995). (More details are provided in Chapters 7 and 9.) Although the Sloane team's focus is on reducing "disruptive behaviors" during bathing, they provide excellent examples of ways to modify the interpersonal and physical environments to create a positive context for bathing. This is important because functional performance is highly influenced by context. Step-by-step guidelines entitled "Family Information for Bathing a Patient with Alzheimer's Disease at Home" are available on the Internet at the Alzheimer's Disease On-Line Learning Center of the Boston University Alzheimer's Disease Center (*www.visn1.org/Alzheimer*).[1]

## Dressing

Dressing is the ADL that has been studied the most extensively. A dressing assessment protocol (Beck, 1988; Heacock et al., 1997) and a supportive behavioral intervention known as SPID ("Strategies to Promote Independence in Dressing"; Beck et al., 1992, 1997) have been developed for nursing facility residents with cognitive impairment. A significant improvement in dressing performance was achieved by more than 75% of the residents studied when trained nursing assistants implemented SPID. More than 20% of residents reached their maximum intervention effect during the first week, and another 30% achieved maximum effect after Week 5 or 6 of the study. Thorough assessment was suggested as a way to distinguish individuals who simply need the opportunity to dress themselves from those who need retraining to improve their dressing performance (Beck et al., 1997). Use of the dressing assessment facilitates clinical decision making by matching the type, amount, and timing of assistance to the particular level of function. This principle can be applied to any ADL.

## Toileting/Continence

A task analysis of the steps that are involved in toileting and identification of the multiple factors influencing continence has been conducted (Hutchinson et al., 1996). Following the prototype that was described for dressing, an algorithm can be developed to match the appropriate level and type of caregiver assistance with a care recipient's needs to perform the toileting task components competently.

---

[1]Also available is the Sloane team's videotape, *Solving Bathing Problems in Persons with Alzheimer's Disease and Related Dementias,* which can be ordered from Health Professions Press.

Mrs. Ewing independently recognizes the urge to void. With a verbal prompt, she walks to the bathroom, but she requires a nonverbal prompt (gesture) to close the door and pull down her pants. She sits and voids without assistance, but she requires help to wipe herself with toilet tissue and to stand up from the toilet.

Additional interventions for toileting difficulties include the following (Hutchinson et al., 1996):

- Behavioral interventions such as habit training (timed voiding) and prompted voiding; these require verbal prompting and reminders in the early stages of dementia and toileting schedules during normal voiding times in the later stages of dementia
- Establish a routine.
- Clothing modification (e.g., "pull-on" pants with elastic waistband, Velcro closures in lieu of shoelaces)
- Assisting with bathroom location
- Watching for cues that indicate a person's need to use the bathroom
- Becoming familiar with clients (e.g., observing toileting patterns, interpreting behavior, choosing successful strategies)
- Preserving dignity (e.g., respecting privacy, minimizing embarrassment by whispering, behaving naturally)
- Physical assistance and cognitive assistance (e.g., providing directions, pointing to toilet)

## Eating

The ability to plan and prepare meals, which are IADLs, is affected in the early stages of dementia. The Eating Behavior Scale includes six behaviors for the PADL of eating: initiation, maintain attention, location of all foods, correct use of utensils, safety, and termination (Tully et al., 1997). The type of assistance required is rated as "independent," "needing verbal prompts," "needing physical assistance," and "total assistance."

In a study of factors that influence eating in nursing facility units that accommodate residents with cognitive impairment, nearly all of the residents needed to be encouraged to eat, required assistance with their meals, or had to be fed, yet staffing was not adequate to meet these needs (Kayser-Jones & Schell, 1997). Two strategies that arose from this study are recommended here (approaches to eating/feeding are included in Chapter 10): 1) encourage independence while providing supervision and assistance and 2) create a social mealtime environment and simplify the eating process.

# REFERENCES

American Psychiatric Association. (1994). *Diagnostic and statistical manual of mental disorders* (4th ed.). Washington, DC: American Psychiatric Press.

Beck, C. (1988). Measurement of dressing performance in persons with dementia. *American Journal of Alzheimer Care and Related Disorders and Research, 3,* 21–25.

Beck, C.K., & Frank, L.B. (1997). Assessing functioning and self-care abilities in Alzheimer disease research. *Alzheimer Disease and Associated Disorders, 11*(Suppl. 6), 73–80.

Beck, C., Heacock, P., & Mercer, S. (Producers). (1992). *The resident with dementia: Strategies to promote independence in dressing* [Videocassette]. Baltimore: University of Maryland at Baltimore Video Press.

Beck, C., Heacock, P., Mercer, S.O., Walls, R.C., Rapp, C.G., & Vogelpohl, R.S. (1997). Improving dressing behavior in cognitively impaired nursing home residents. *Nursing Research, 46,* 126–132.

Bennett, J.A. (1999). Activities of daily living: Old-fashioned or still useful? *Journal of Gerontological Nursing, 25*(5), 22–29.

Burgener, S.C., Jirovec, M., Murrell, L., & Barton, D. (1992). Caregiver and environmental variables related to difficult behaviors in institutionalized, demented elderly persons. *Journal of Gerontology, 47,* P242–P249.

Burns, R., Mortimer, J.A., & Merchak, P. (1994). Cognitive performance test: A new approach to functional assessment in Alzheimer's disease. *Journal of Geriatric Psychiatry and Neurology, 7,* 46–54.

Burns, T., Hepburn, K., Maddox, M., & Smith, S. (1998). *Alzheimer's caregiving strategies* [CD-ROM]. Minneapolis: Healthcare Interactive, Inc.

Cohen-Mansfield, J., Werner, P., & Reisberg, B. (1995). Temporal order of cognitive and functional loss in a nursing home population. *Journal of the American Geriatrics Society, 43,* 974–978.

Diehl, M., Marsiske, M., Horgas, A.L., & Saczynski, J. (1998). *Psychometric properties of the Revised Observed Tasks of Daily Living.* Poster presented at the 51st Annual Scientific Meeting of the Gerontological Society of America, November 20–24, 1998, Philadelphia.

Gallo, J.J., Reichel, W., & Andersen, L.M. (1995). *Handbook of geriatric assessment* (2nd ed.). Gaithersburg, MD: Aspen Publishers.

Heacock, P., Beck, C., Souder, E., & Mercer, S. (1997). Assessing dressing ability in dementia. *Geriatric Nursing, 18*(3), 107–111.

Hutchinson, S., Leger-Krall, S., & Wilson, H.S. (1996). Toileting: A biobehavioral challenge in Alzheimer's dementia care. *Journal of Gerontological Nursing, 22*(10), 18–27.

Karagiozis, J. (1998). Direct assessment of functional abilities. *Gerontologist, 38,* 113–121.

Kayser-Jones, J. (1997). Inadequate staffing at mealtime: Implications for nursing and health policy. *Journal of Gerontological Nursing, 23*(8), 14–21.

Kayser-Jones, J., & Schell, E. (1997). The mealtime experience of a cognitively impaired elder: Ineffective and effective strategies. *Journal of Gerontological Nursing, 23*(7), 33–39.

Lawton, M.P. (1983). Environment and other determinants of well being in older people. *Gerontologist, 23,* 349–357.

Lawton, M.P., & Brody, E. (1969). Assessment of older people: Self-maintaining and instrumental activities of daily living. *Gerontologist, 9,* 170–186.

Leidy, N.K. (1994). Functional status and the forward progress of merry-go-rounds: Toward a coherent analytical framework. *Nursing Research, 43,* 196–202.

Morris, J.N., Fries, B.E., Steel, K., Ikegami, N., Bernabei, R., Carpenter, I., Gilgen, R., Hirdes, J.P., & Topinkova, E. (1997). Comprehensive clinical assessment in community setting: Applicability of the MDS-HC. *Journal of the American Geriatrics Society, 45,* 1017–1024.

Morris, J.N., Hawes, C., Murphy, K., Nonemaker, S., Phillips, C., Fries, B.E., & Mor, V. (1990). *Resident assessment instrument training manual and resource guide.* Natick, MA: Eliot Press.

Morris, J.N., Mahoney, E.K., Murphy, K.N., Gornstein, E.S., Ruchlin, H.S., & Lipsitz, L.A. (1998). A randomized controlled nursing intervention to maintain functional status in nursing home residents. *Canadian Journal of Quality in Health Care, 14*(3), 14–22.

Morris, J.N., Nonemaker, S., Murphy, K., Hawes, C., Fries, B.E., Mor, V., & Phillips, C. (1997). A commitment to change: Revision of HCFA's RAI. *Journal of the American Geriatrics Society, 45,* 1011–1016.

National Citizens Coalition for Nursing Home Reform. (1986). *A consumer perspective on quality care: The residents' point of view (summary report).* Washington, DC: American Society of Consultant Pharmacists.

Omnibus Budget Reconciliation Act of 1987, PL 100–203, 42 C.F.R. § 483.25 *et seq.*

Sloane, P.D., Rader, J., Barrick, A.-L., Hoeffer, B., Dwyer, S., McKenzie, D., Lavelle, M., Buckwalter, K., Arrington, L., & Pruitt, T. (1995). Bathing persons with dementia. *Gerontologist, 35,* 672–678.

Spector, W.D. (1997). Measuring functioning in daily activities for persons with dementia. *Alzheimer Disease and Associated Disorders, 11*(Suppl. 6), 81–90.

Stehman, J.M., Strachan, G.I., Glenner, J.A., Glenner, G.G., & Neubauer, J.K. (1996). *Handbook of dementia care.* Baltimore: The Johns Hopkins University Press.

Stone, J.R., Wyman, J.F., & Salisbury, S.A. (1999). *Clinical gerontological nursing: A guide to advanced practice* (2nd ed.). Philadelphia: W.B. Saunders.

Tappen, R.M. (1994). Development of the Refined ADL Assessment Scale for patients with Alzheimer's and related disorders. *Journal of Gerontological Nursing, 20*(6), 36–42.

Trudeau, S.A. (1999). Prevention of physical impairment in persons with advanced Alzheimer's disease. In L. Volicer & L. Bloom-Charette (Eds.), *Enhancing the quality of life in advanced dementia* (pp. 80–90). Philadelphia: Brunner/Mazel.

Tully, M.W., Matrakas, K.L., Muir, J., & Musallam, K. (1997). The Eating Behavior Scale: A simple method of assessing functional ability in patients with Alzheimer's disease. *Journal of Gerontological Nursing, 23*(7), 9–15.

# 6

# Inability to Initiate Meaningful Activities

The inability to initiate meaningful activities, although easy to overlook, affects both people with dementia and their caregivers. This inability has roots in functional impairment and depression, and its effects are far reaching. Lack of meaningful activity may result in negative states such as apathy or agitation for people with dementia and in frustration and burden for caregivers (Volicer, Hurley, & Mahoney, 1995). Conversely, involvement with meaningful activity is important for the maintenance of functional abilities, social involvement, provision of a feeling of success and accomplishment, improvement in mood, and reduction of disruptive behaviors (Kovach & Henschel, 1996; Teri & Logsdon, 1991).

People with dementia live in the moment, and there is widespread agreement among experts that the moment should be pleasurable. In fact, one of the primary goals when working with people with dementia is the maintenance of quality of life and pleasure (Omnibus Budget Reconciliation Act, 1987). Intervention goals for people with the inability to initiate meaningful activity, therefore, are to prevent excess disability and to improve their interaction with the environment and their quality of life.

Fred Franklin is an 80-year-old retired chef. He and his wife Fran sold their house and moved into a one-bedroom apartment in an assisted living facility 2 years ago when Fred was first diagnosed as having Alzheimer's disease. This arrangement has been good because they feel free from worries about maintaining a house. Fran is especially appreciative for the 30 minutes a day when Fred receives help from the home health aide, because it gives her a break from the otherwise constant attention that Fred requires. For most of the day, Fred follows Fran around. She jokingly tells her friends, "He's like a shadow," but actually his behavior annoys Fran, who feels she has no space and no privacy, even to use the bathroom. Fred no longer cooks, but repeatedly asks, "What are we having for dinner? Is it time to eat?" Her answers pacify him for a couple of minutes, but then he asks again. He mirrors her moves around the kitchen, from refrigerator to sink to stove and back. Fran confides to the nurse in the assisted living facility's health center that her husband is "driving her crazy," and she wonders why he cannot find something to do.

The inability to initiate meaningful activities includes but also goes beyond the nursing diagnosis "diversional activity deficit," which Gordon defined as "decreased engagement in recreational or leisure activities" (1997, p. 217). It is different in that 1) the person with dementia may not be able to report boredom or express a wish for something to do; 2) clinical indicators are more often behavioral than verbal; and 3) meaningful activity may include recreational/leisure pursuits but is broader in that it is therapeutic and includes daily activities that are more than just diversional. The Alzheimer's Association (2000) defined activities as "the things we do. ... They can represent who we are and what we're about" (p. 1). Usual activities cannot be undertaken, not only because there is a lack of opportunity but also because cognitive and physical functional impairments alter the capacity of people with dementia to communicate, engage in activity, and experience and respond to various types of stimulation (Kovach & Magliocco, 1998).

People with dementia who are unable to initiate meaningful activities may be unoccupied and appear bored or not engaged with the environment, sitting motionless or wandering around aimlessly. They spend more time in a state of inner retreat, and this withdrawn behavior may manifest itself as lack of behavior, somnolence, perseveration, or nondirected verbal agitation (Kovach & Magliocco, 1998). For example, Mr. Franklin follows his wife around, shadows her movements, and asks repetitive questions, as if wondering where to go or what to do.

The inability to initiate meaningful activities is rooted in the core symptoms of functional impairment and depression, the physical and social environment, and the overall health of the person with dementia. These risk factors and their relationships are depicted in the model of behavioral symptoms of dementia presented in the Introduction. The person with the inability to initiate meaningful activities still can have the energy and desire to do things but lack the ability to organize, plan, initiate, and successfully complete even simple activities because of functional impairment (Alzheimer's Association, 2000). Depression can result in loss of interest and energy, as described in Chapter 3.

General health status also is important. For example, fatigue or activity intolerance, stemming from disease or disuse and inactivity, can reduce the energy available for an activity. Hearing and vision also may play a role. A study of the effects of hearing impairments on nursing facility residents revealed a strong association between hearing impairments and low levels of social engagement and little or no time spent in activities (Resnick, Fries, & Verbrugge, 1997). If leisure activities preferred by the older adult require good visual skills, such as with reading, sewing, or needlework, then the older adult may become bored and withdrawn when vision changes interfere with these endeavors (Miller, 1999).

The inability to initiate meaningful activities may be a natural part of the progression of dementia or it may result from social, environmental, and sensory deprivation (Kovach & Magliocco, 1998). What constitutes a meaningful activity varies not only by severity of disease but also by life history and preferences. Older adults in general are apt to engage in an activity that they perceive to be meaningful. For people with dementia, task complexity needs to be considered in relation to the functional level of the individual. Activities that are too difficult can lead to frustration and avoidance. Activities that are infantilizing or that the person views as childish may have a negative effect on self-esteem and engagement.

## BEHAVIOR MANAGEMENT STRATEGIES

The goal of treatment is to create an environment with optimum stimulation and a steady flow of meaningful activities within the functional capacity of the person. People with functional impairment need structured activities that employ previously learned motor patterns (Beck, Modlin, Heithoff, & Shue, 1992). One component of an activity program is organized therapeutic activity. In addition, a "lifestyle approach" has been developed that uses assessment, programming, and therapeutic environment to establish a daily routine that is familiar and fills people's days with meaningful activities (Simard, 1999). Activities are planned on a one-to-one basis or as group programs. One-to-one activities are useful for people whose attention is difficult to maintain and provide intimate, private time to build relationships. Group activities promote socialization and a sense of belonging (Alzheimer's Association, 2000). In a study of participation in therapeutic activities, Kovach and

Magliocco (1998) found that even when a group is gathered, the therapeutic activity is designed as a one-to-one interaction.

## GUIDELINES FOR CHOOSING ACTIVITIES

Planning meaningful activities begins with an assessment of the person, which includes the individual's medical history, history of interests and habits, severity of functional impairments, and emotional state and behavior (Alzheimer's Association, 2000; Stehman, Strachan, Glenner, Glenner, & Neubauer, 1996). The assessment must be updated as the person's level of functional impairment changes to maintain a match between abilities and activities. Examples of areas to assess include the following:

* What skills and abilities does the person retain?
* What is the degree of functional impairment (see Chapters 2 and 5)?
* Does the person have physical health problems (e.g., arthritis, hearing impairment)?
* What does the person enjoy doing?

The Pleasant Events Schedule-Alzheimer's Disease (PES-AD) (Logsdon & Teri, 1997; Teri & Logsdon, 1991) was developed to help both professional and family caregivers identify those activities that are enjoyable to individuals with dementia. The revised Short PES-AD includes 20 activities that people with dementia may enjoy. Caregivers, together with the older adult when possible, rate each of the items for frequency and perceived enjoyability. Besides its usefulness as an assessment tool, the list of activities offers an easy-to-use compendium of ideas for pleasant activities, particularly for people in early to moderate stages of dementia.

> Mr. and Mrs. Franklin sat down together and completed the Short PES-AD given to them by the health center nurse. As Fran read the activities, she found a few that Fred does often—walking, being outside, and watching basketball games—even if it is for only a few minutes at a time. She also found activities that Fred used to enjoy—working in the yard, talking about his restaurant, and making snacks. She plans to include more of these activities in his day. With the nurse's guidance, Fran realized that she had been viewing "activity" as a separate event and had been feeling stressed that planning such events seemed like "just one more thing to do."
>
> After discussing the completed PES-AD and reading the activity programming suggestions on the Alzheimer's Association website, Fran tried the "lifestyle approach" to establish a daily routine that gives structure to the day and involves Fred in more activities. In the morning, he

helps her prepare a simple breakfast and they discuss the newspaper before he washes up, shaves with an electric razor, and brushes his teeth. Fred then walks to the corner mailbox to mail letters, comes home, and reads his own mail with Fran. Together, they prepare and eat lunch, then clear and wash the dishes. In the afternoon, Fred works in the garden or rakes leaves or looks at photographs and puts them in piles. He likes to look through recipe books that picture the food, which reminds him of his days as a chef. At dinnertime, he collects food from the refrigerator or cabinet, peels vegetables, and sets the table. He loves to fold the napkins into creative shapes. After dinner, he and Fran take a walk or watch an old movie. He brushes the dog before getting ready for bed. The day is pretty full and he seems to enjoy it. Even though Fran needs to help him get started with most of the activities, once started he can continue and keep involved for about 20 minutes or more at a time.

General guidelines, which are applicable to all activities, are presented in Table 6.1. Some activities (e.g., exercise, music) can be adapted for use across all stages of dementia, whereas others are more stage specific. Simple and innovative behavioral interventions are described according to the stage of dementia for which they may be most useful. Choice of an intervention should be based on the person's assessment, including functional capacity and enjoyment, and on the goals of meaningful activity—preventing excess disability, providing sensory stimulation, and promoting quality of life.

**Table 6.1.    Guidelines for planning activities for people with dementia**

| Principle | Rationale |
| --- | --- |
| Focus on enjoyment, not achievement | The goals of a therapeutic program are to prevent excess disability and help the person "feel good."<br>Meaningful activities must be voluntary. |
| Create "failure-free" environment | Helps person maintain self-esteem |
| Design therapeutic activities to stimulate multiple senses | The ability to experience a range of human responses (emotions, behavior) continues across mild, moderate, and severe stages of dementia. |
| Make activities part of daily routine | Maintains home-like routines<br>It is not possible to have planned activities for an entire day. Routine activities are done anyway.<br>Not an extra burden for the caregiver |
| Plan structured activities that employ previously learned motor patterns | These tasks require no new learning, yet can make the person feel useful and productive. |

*Sources:* Alzheimer's Association (2000), Simard (1999), and Stehman et al. (1996).

## MANAGEMENT STRATEGIES FOR
## EARLY TO MODERATE STAGES OF DEMENTIA

There are several interventions for people in early to moderate stages of dementia: cognitive activities, functional household activities, diversional activities, reminiscence, Video Respite®, and exercise.

### Cognitive Activities

Carefully planned cognitive remediation, targeted to remaining abilities, can slow the rate of decline in functional performance in people with dementia (Quayhagen, Quayhagen, Corbeil, Roth, & Rodgers, 1995). Quayhagen and associates found that skills in problem-solving tasks, such as planning activities and dealing with practical problems, could be taught to people with mild to moderate decline in cognitive function. These skills depend on retained procedural learning and interpersonal skills rather than the ability to learn something new, which may already have been lost. In this experimental study, memory techniques, both verbal and visual, were focused on the mental functions of recall and recognition. Family members were taught active cognitive stimulation exercises that they carried out at home for 3 months. Care recipients in the experimental group initially improved in cognitive and behavioral performance with treatment but returned to their former level of functioning by the ninth month of the study. In contrast, the control group either remained static or declined on these variables.

The goal of cognitive stimulation is to eliminate excess disability. Careful assessment is necessary to plan activities that maximize remaining skills, capitalize on strengths and needs, and minimize or avoid areas of weakness (Stehman et al., 1996).

Examples of cognitive activities (Alzheimer's Association, 2000; Dowling, 1995; Silverio & Koenig-Coste, 1999; Stehman et al., 1996) include

- Doing jigsaw puzzles—modified to abilities
- Reading magazines to maintain long-established interests
- Participating in reminiscence activities to stimulate long-term memory
- Playing cards
- Playing word games—trivia, crossword puzzles, cognitive stimulation
- Having a conversation about a topic of interest or current events
- Reading and writing poetry
- Painting

### Functional Household Activities

Daily housekeeping tasks are good for people with dementia because no new learning is required, yet participation can make them feel useful and productive. Caregivers should simplify these activities if necessary or arrange for their care recipients to participate in only some of the steps.

> Fred has always loved to cook. Although he is no longer able to plan and prepare a full meal, he is able to participate and enjoys this activity. Fran involves him in the planning when she can. For example, she asks, "Are mashed potatoes okay? We're having fish and salad." Fran sets out the potatoes and peeler and asks Fred to peel the potatoes. She asks him to wash them, then cut them in half. After peeling the first potato, Fred becomes distracted and asks, "What should I do?" Fran replies, "Please peel the potato on the counter."

Examples of other functional household activities (Alzheimer's Association, 2000; Miller, Peckhan, & Peckman, 1995; Silverio & Koenig-Coste, 1999; Stehman et al., 1996) include

- Folding laundry
- Raking leaves
- Gardening—indoors and outdoors
- Sweeping and dusting
- Clearing and setting tables
- Making beds
- Planning and going on a shopping trip
- Preparing meals (one dish, with steps presented one at a time by the caregiver)

## Diversional Activities

Recreational activities make positive use of leisure time. In addition, activities can be used as a way to divert people with dementia from difficult situations. For example, an invitation to have a cup of tea may distract a person who is intent on leaving the house or facility (Alzheimer's Association, 2000).

Examples of diversional activities (Alzheimer's Association, 2000; Silverio & Koenig-Coste, 1999; Stehman et al., 1996; Teri & Logsdon, 1991) include

- Photography
- Videotaping
- Watching or participating in sports
- Participating in community outreach—soup kitchens, volunteer opportunities
- Going for a ride

## Reminiscence

Reminiscence is the process of recalling the past and, as such, uses preserved long-term memory, which often is a strength of the person with dementia. Arruda (1999) poignantly referred to reminiscence as a "trip back to a safer era." Reminiscence can be silent or spoken, solitary or interactional, or spontaneous or structured (Burnside, 1990). The general therapeutic benefits of reminiscence for older adults have been documented in research studies and clinical reports. Several examples of the use of reminiscence for people with dementia show that it can be used effectively with them.

Reminiscence activities can be done individually or in a group setting. Sometimes props are used, for example, "memory boxes" or "theme boxes" in which items representing a theme are collected. Group reminiscence might focus on a common theme as well, such as familiar music or "how I met my spouse." Individual reminiscence is based on particular knowledge of the person. An approach for people in the early stage of dementia is to have the person keep a journal of things that are important to him or her. The journal can be used for later reference. As cognitive and language function decline, the person's family members can be interviewed to elicit happy memories.

## Video Respite®[1]

Video Respite® is an innovative intervention that uses videotapes created specifically for people with dementia to capture and maintain their attention, enabling caregivers to enjoy respite time (Lund, Hi, Caserta, & Wright, 1995). Several tapes have been developed that use a "friendly visitor" who talks and asks question about familiar things such as parents, growing up, babies, pets, and holidays. Pauses are interspersed to give viewers an opportunity to respond. The videotapes also include singing and simple exercises. Both individualized and generic videotapes have been developed that attempt to tap a wide range of life experiences and cultural perspectives. Although this intervention is still being tested, the evaluations gathered by the research team report positive results, including attentiveness, verbal response, and enjoyment (Lund et al., 1995). The researchers also report that the tapes may be too simple for some people in the early stage of dementia, who appear to be embarrassed if others know that they are responding to the tapes.

## Exercise

Physical exercise improves the physiological health of elderly people by reducing weight, blood pressure, blood sugar, and cholesterol; decreasing the risk of cardiovascular disease and falls; and maintaining bone density. Lack of

[1]Several tapes in the Video Respite® series are available from Health Professions Press, 888-337-8808 or www.healthpropress.com.

exercise results in disuse syndrome ("if you don't use it, you lose it"). Exercise also improves the mental health of older adults by increasing feelings of well-being, energy, and accomplishment (Emery & Blumenthal, 1990). Although all older adults benefit from regular exercise, it is especially important for people with dementia. In a review of research that addressed exercise as an intervention for people with dementia, Beck and colleagues (1990) concluded that exercise decreases disruptive behaviors, increases oxygen perfusion to the brain, improves social skills such as initiating conversation and displaying common courtesies, and provides an acceptable replacement for the repetitive movements that are common in people with dementia. People with dementia need physical exercise that uses previously learned motor patterns (Beck et al., 1992). Examples include planned walking, dancing, moving rhythmically to music, and stretching exercises (Weaver, 1995).

## MANAGEMENT STRATEGIES FOR
## MODERATE TO LATE STAGES OF DEMENTIA

There are several interventions for people in moderate to late stages of dementia: simulated presence therapy, music, Bright Eyes, reminiscence, animal-assisted therapy, Merry Walker, and Snoezelen.

### Simulated Presence Therapy

Simulated presence therapy (SPT) employs a personalized audiotape that uses preserved long-term memories (Camberg et al., 1999; Woods & Ashley, 1995). Families are interviewed to collect information such as favorite songs and poems, happy memories, and important events from the past. An audiotape is created that provides a one-sided conversation with strategic pauses in the tape to allow for a response by the person with dementia. This intervention is similar to Video Respite except that SPT uses an autoreverse tape recorder that is placed in a fanny pack and a head-set, making the intervention portable. SPT has been used for people who are agitated as well as those who are withdrawn, and its use has resulted in improved behavior (Camberg et al., 1999).

### Music

The therapeutic effects of music have received significant attention in practice and the literature. Music is used to increase alertness, encourage movement, reduce agitation, relieve stress, and promote relaxation in both people with dementia and their caregivers, and it provides inclusion and involvement, facilitates communication, fosters creative self-expression, and promotes reminiscence (Brotons, Koger, & Pickett-Cooper, 1997; Casby & Holm, 1994; Clair, 1996; Gerdner, 1997; Goddaer & Abraham, 1994; Ragneskog, Kihlgren, Karlsson, & Norberg, 1996; Tabloski, McKinnon-Howe, & Remington, 1995).

The literature recommends favorite music most highly; therefore, determining the person's music preferences must be part of the assessment. Other types of music that are reported to have positive effects include familiar music and classical music, which has a relaxing effect. Based on a review of the literature, we recommend favorite music for individual activities (e.g., bathing) and familiar or classical music for group activities (e.g., meals, recreation therapy events). In recreation therapy events in which more than one individual is involved, music that was popular for a cohort might be considered, for example, big band music or show tunes from the 1940s and 1950s.

The timing, length, and frequency of music intervention also need to be planned. Some issues to consider include the reason that the music is being used and the expected outcome. For example, Gerdner (1997) suggested that music as an intervention for agitation is most effective when it is implemented before the peak level of agitation. This makes sense and is analogous to what is known about the effective use of pain medication—that more effective pain management is achieved when analgesics are given before pain peaks. When music is used to achieve positive outcomes such as movement, communication, or reminiscence, the length and frequency of treatments are important (Brotons et al., 1997). Research that addresses these issues is ongoing. In the interim, documentation should include target behaviors (e.g., stress, agitation, interaction, movement), specific music interventions (e.g., name of piece, when played), and outcomes achieved.

## Bright Eyes

Bright Eyes is a group activity, organized around a theme, that stimulates all of the senses. An example of a Bright Eyes session, organized around a baseball theme, that was developed at the Edith Nourse Rogers Memorial Veterans Hospital in Bedford, Massachusetts (Trudeau, 1999a) is shown in Table 6.2. Another theme that could be developed into a Bright Eyes protocol is laundry. As described by Stehman and colleagues (1996), hanging wash on an old-fashioned clothesline employs fresh air, fresh-smelling clothes, and the motor (kinesthetic) stimulation of bending and reaching. The wet clothes and clothespins provide the tactile component; clothes blowing in the breeze is the visual component. Outdoor sounds or singing a song lyric such as, "This is the way we do our wash, so early in the morning," and a glass of lemonade or iced tea round out the complete sensory package.

## Reminiscence

Reminiscence has been used with people even in the late stages of dementia with positive results, including increased eye contact, vocalization, relaxation, and signs of connecting with the environment (Kovach & Magliocco, 1998; Mahoney et al., 1999). Pleasant memories are collected through family inter-

*Table 6.2.    Example of Bright Eyes—baseball theme*

| Sense stimulated | Activity |
| --- | --- |
| Olfactory | Freshly cut grass |
| Kinesthetic | Baseball toss |
| Tactile | Felt baseball cap |
| Visual | Picture of baseball field |
| Auditory | Sing "Take Me Out to the Ballgame" |
| Gustatory | Nonalcoholic beer |

From Trudeau S.A. (1999a). Bright Eyes: A structured sensory stimulation intervention. In L. Volicer & L. Bloom-Charette (Eds.), *Enhancing quality of life for persons with advanced Alzheimer's disease* (pp. 93–106). Philadelphia: Brunner/Mazel; reprinted by permission.

views or questionnaires, which is similar to the process described for SPT. Besides the positive outcomes of reminiscence for people with dementia, the process of collecting the memories gives family members a concrete, positive way of contributing to the quality of life of their loved one. Nursing staff report that using reminiscence with people who are in the advanced stages of dementia is more challenging because the interaction may seem more one-sided, but it is beneficial in that it allows them to "know the person" as an individual (Mahoney et al., 1999).

## Animal-Assisted Therapy

In animal-assisted, or pet, therapy animals are used as a therapeutic catalyst (Miller, 1999). The animal may live "in residence" or may be a visitor. Numerous clinical reports document the ability of animals to help fulfill a person's need to love and be loved, help restore emotional equilibrium, enhance self-image and identity, and alleviate depression (Miller, 1999). Animals also stimulate multiple senses, for example, auditory (e.g., birds), tactile, and kinesthetic (e.g., petting a dog). Programs are available in local communities, including pet visitors and pet adoption (e.g., "Adopt a Greyhound" programs).

## Merry Walker

Walking is important in its own right, and it encourages other activities and decreases potential complications from immobility. People with advanced dementia are at risk for difficulties with walking. For example, neuromuscular changes or medication side effects such as tardive dyskinesia result in an unsteady gait and scissoring. Immobility from any cause (e.g., illness, restraints) results in deconditioning and contractures. People with dementia who have been in bed for long periods of time actually forget how to walk. The Merry Walker is an assistive device that facilitates safe walking for people with advanced dementia. It combines the stability of a walker with a seat that allows people to sit down if tired (Trudeau, 1999b).

## Snoezelen

Snoezelen (pronounced "snooze-lin") is a multisensory environment program that was designed for people with severe learning disabilities and sensory deficits and has been used more recently for people with dementia. The program, which literally means "sniff and doze," combines a comfortable, secure environment with stimulation of the senses (Pinkney & Barker, 1994). This is accomplished by using a combination of soft music, aromatic oils, and gentle light filtered through an oil-filled wheel to project moving colored images. Snoezelen has been used at the Edith Nourse Rogers Memorial Veterans Hospital in Bedford, Massachusetts, for relaxation and for sensory stimulation in people with advanced dementia (Volicer, Mahoney, & Brown, 1998). This intervention provides a wide range of sensory experiences that improve the quality of life of people with dementia. The greatest asset of Snoezelen lies in its capacity to provide meaningful activity without requiring intellectual reasoning or verbal responses. This asset enables participants to engage at whatever level is appropriate for them, resulting in a release of stress and frustration.

## DOCUMENTING RESPONSES TO INTERVENTIONS

Resident participation in activity programs must be recorded in nursing facilities. Care plans must reflect the residents' involvement in the daily programming, and progress notes should reflect the actual involvement of each resident (Simard, 1999). Positive outcomes may include increased independence, decreased behavioral symptoms, or improved psychological well-being, evidenced by behaviors such as happier mood, participation in activities, or more positive interaction with family or staff. Simard also reported anecdotal evidence of increased family satisfaction with visits and quality of care when comprehensive activity programs have been implemented. Also, it is possible that actual outcomes for individuals will not be positive, for example, if planned activities are either infantilizing or too complex. Documentation of resident response allows for program adjustment.

A simple, objective way to measure a person's participation, described by Kovach and Henschel (1996, p. 37), is to observe the person every 3 minutes and code participation as "active," "passive," "null," "dozing," or "unrelated." They also suggested that the "ability to make a cognitive tie" to an activity is an important predictor of active involvement in an activity.

Jennings (1999, p. 95) argued that "human flourishing, personal agency, human relationships, and meaningful interaction" are key elements of quality of life for people with dementia. Each of these outcomes has been linked with meaningful activity. Therefore, an individualized plan of care that facilitates the person's active involvement in meaningful activities across the continuum of the disease is critical to both quality of care and quality of life.

## REFERENCES

Alzheimer's Association. (2000). *Activity-based Alzheimer's care* [On-line]. Available: www.alz.org/nc/qcare/activity.htm

Arruda, R. (1999). *Lollipops for Esther—Enter her world.* Paper presented at the Quality of Life for Persons with Dementia meeting, March 31, 1999, Bedford, MA.

Beck, C., Modlin, R., Heithoff, K., & Shue, V. (1992). Exercise as an intervention for behavior problems. *Geriatric Nursing, 13*(5), 273–275.

Brotons, M., Koger, S.M., & Pickett-Cooper, P. (1997). Music and dementia: A review of literature. *Journal of Music Therapy, 34,* 204–245.

Burnside, I. (1990). Reminiscence: An independent nursing intervention for the elderly. *Issues in Mental Health Nursing, 11,* 33–48.

Camberg, L., Woods, P., Ooi, W.L., Hurley, A., Volicer, L., Ashley, J., Odenheimer, G., & McIntyre, K. (1999). Evaluation of simulated presence: A personalized approach to enhance well being in persons with Alzheimer's disease. *Journal of the American Geriatrics Society, 47,* 446–452.

Casby, J.A., & Holm, M.B. (1994). The effect of music on repetitive disruptive vocalizations of persons with dementia. *American Journal of Occupational Therapy, 48,* 883–889.

Clair, A.A. (1996). *Therapeutic uses of music with older adults.* Baltimore: Health Professions Press.

Dowling, J.R. (1995). Keeping busy: A handbook of activities for persons with dementia. Baltimore: The Johns Hopkins University Press.

Emery, C., & Blumenthal, J. (1990). Perceived change among participants in an exercise program for older adults. *Gerontologist, 30,* 516–521.

Gerdner, L. (1997). An individualized music intervention for agitation. *Journal of the American Psychiatric Nurses Association, 3,* 177–184.

Goddaer, J., & Abraham, I.L. (1994). Effects of relaxing music on agitation during meals among nursing home residents with severe cognitive impairment. *Archives of Psychiatric Nursing, 8*(3), 150–158.

Gordon, M. (1997). *Manual of nursing diagnoses 1997–1998.* St. Louis: Mosby.

Jennings, B. (1999). A life greater than the sum of its sensations: Ethics, dementia, and the quality of life. *Journal of Mental Health and Aging, 5*(1), 95–106.

Kovach, C.R., & Henschel, H. (1996). Planning activities for patients with dementia: A descriptive study of therapeutic activities on special care units. *Journal of Gerontological Nursing, 22*(9), 33–38.

Kovach, C.R., & Magliocco, J.S. (1998). Late-stage dementia and participation in therapeutic activities. *Applied Nursing Research, 11*(4), 167–173.

Logsdon, R.G., & Teri, L. (1997). The Pleasant Events Schedule–AD: Psychometric properties and relationship to depression and cognition in Alzheimer's disease patients. *Gerontologist, 37,* 40–45.

Lund, D.A., Hi, R.D., Caserta, M.S., & Wright, S.D. (1995). Video Respite: An innovative resource for family, professional caregivers, and persons with dementia. *Gerontologist, 35,* 683–687.

Mahoney, E.K., Bose, S., Barron, A.M., Stafford, K., Harvey, R., Hurley, A.C., & Volicer, L. (1999). *Reminiscence during bathing persons with dementia: Perspectives of patient, nurse and family.* Unpublished manuscript, Geriatric Research, Education and Clinical Center, Edith Nourse Rogers Memorial Veterans Hospital, Bedford, MA.

Miller, C.A. (1999). *Nursing care of older adults* (3rd ed.). Philadelphia: Lippincott.

Miller, M.E., Peckhan, C.W., & Peckman, A.B. (1995). *Activities keep me going & going.* Vol. 2. Centerville, OH: Marco Printed Products.

Omnibus Budget Reconciliation Act of 1987, PL 101-203, 42 C.F.R. § 483 *et seq.*

Pinkney, L., & Barker, P. (1994). "Snoezelen"—An evaluation of a sensory environment used by people who are elderly and confused. In R. Hutchinson & J. Kewin (Eds.), *Sensations & disability* (pp. 172–183). Chesterfield, UK: ROMPA.

Quayhagen, M.P., Quayhagen, M., Corbeil, R.R., Roth, P., & Rodgers, J.A. (1995). A dyadic remediation program for care recipients with dementia. *Nursing Research, 44,* 153–159.

Ragneskog, H., Kihlgren, M., Karlsson, I., & Norberg, A. (1996). Dinner music for demented patients. *Clinical Nursing Research, 5,* 262–282.

Resnick, H.E., Fries, B.E., & Verbrugge, L.M. (1997). Windows to their world: The effect of sensory impairments on social engagement and activity time in nursing home residents. *Journals of Gerontology, Series B: Psychological Sciences and Social Sciences, 52,* S135–S144.

Silverio, E., & Koenig-Coste, J. (1999). *Activities for persons with early stage Alzheimer's disease.* Conference materials distributed at the Quality of Life for Persons with Dementia meeting, March 31, 1999, Bedford, MA.

Simard, J. (1999). Making a positive difference in the lives of nursing home residents with Alzheimer's disease: The lifestyle approach. *Alzheimer Disease and Associated Disorders, 13*(Suppl. 1), S67–S72.

Stehman, J.M., Strachan, G.I., Glenner, J.A., Glenner, G.G., & Neubauer, J.K. (1996). *Handbook of dementia care.* Baltimore: The Johns Hopkins University Press.

Tabloski, P., McKinnon-Howe, L., & Remington, R. (1995). Effects of calming music on the level of agitation in cognitively impaired nursing home residents. *American Journal of Alzheimer's Care and Related Disorders and Research, 10*(1), 10–15.

Teri, L., & Logsdon, R.G. (1991). Identifying pleasant activities for Alzheimer's disease patients: The Pleasant Events Schedule-AD. *Gerontologist, 31,* 124–127.

Trudeau, S.A. (1999a). Bright Eyes: A structured sensory stimulation intervention. In L. Volicer & L. Bloom-Charette (Eds.), *Enhancing quality of life for persons with advanced Alzheimer's disease* (pp. 93–106). Philadelphia: Brunner/Mazel.

Trudeau, S.A. (1999b). Prevention of physical limitations in advanced Alzheimer's disease. In L. Volicer & L. Bloom-Charette (Eds.), *Enhancing quality of life for persons with advanced Alzheimer's disease* (pp. 80–90). Philadelphia: Brunner/Mazel.

Volicer, L., Hurley, A.C., & Mahoney, E. (1995). Management of behavioral symptoms of dementia. *Nursing Home Medicine, 12*(3), 300–306.

Volicer, L., Mahoney, E., & Brown, E.J. (1998). Nonpharmacological approaches to the management of the behavioral consequences of advanced dementia. In M. Kaplan &

S.B. Hoffman (Eds.), *Behaviors in dementia: Best practices for successful management* (pp. 155–176). Baltimore: Health Professions Press.

Weaver, D. (1995). Activity interventions. In J. Rader & E.M. Tornquist (Eds.), *Individualized dementia care: Creative, compassionate approaches* (pp. 197–207). New York: Springer.

Woods, P., & Ashley, J. (1995). Simulated presence therapy: Using selected memories to manage problem behavior in Alzheimer's disease patients. *Geriatric Nursing, 16*(1), 9–14.

# 7

# Anxiety

Anxiety is defined as a vague, uneasy feeling, the source of which often is non-specific or unknown to the individual who is experiencing it (Gordon, 1997). Anxiety is a feeling of distress, subjectively experienced as fear or worry, and objectively expressed through autonomic and central nervous system responses. Anxiety is distressing and threatens well-being and quality of life. It is both a normal and a pathological emotional response and serves an adaptive purpose in coping with danger or uncertainty (Sussman, 1988). Anxiety may be beneficial when it motivates protective behaviors, but it is detrimental when it channels personal energy into defensive behaviors (Miller, 1999).

## ANXIETY IN OLDER ADULTS

Anxiety is a common human emotion experienced throughout life (Shamoian, 1991). Data on anxiety in the general older adult population are conflicting, with reports on its prevalence ranging from 5% to 68%, depending on the location and nature of the individuals studied, the size of the study sample, and the assessment scales that are used. Anxiety exists in elderly people as a symptom ("state") and as a disorder ("trait"). The presence of anxiety is a negative factor that interferes with performance and increases risk for morbidity from cardiovascular disease (Shamoian, 1991). This conclusion is based on catecholamine studies in anxious older people that demonstrate an elevation of urinary epinephrine levels and heart rate during stress, with a slower return of these parameters to baseline in older adults when compared with younger adults.

## ANXIETY AND DEMENTIA

Anxiety among older people with dementia is a common symptom. The prevalence of anxiety is reported to be 12%–69% in people with dementia (Bolger, Carpenter, & Strauss, 1994; Jost & Grossberg, 1996). This variation probably results from the lack of a consistent approach for defining and measuring anxiety in dementia. In addition, it is possible that the prevalence of anxiety varies across the stages of dementia severity, so that the reported frequency is different depending on the population that is studied. For example, the behavior "appears anxious" occurred at least once weekly in 69% of outpatients with Alzheimer's disease who were rated by their caregivers using the Revised Memory and Behavior Problem Checklist (Logsdon & Teri, 1997). Dementia tends to have an inverse relationship with anxiety, and anxiety is common only in the early stages of dementia (Folks, 1999). This also may be true of "anxiety disorder" (see later in this chapter) and the frequently observed "anxious symptoms" seen later in the course of dementia, any of which may be a response to the core symptoms of functional impairment: depression, delusions, and hallucinations (see the model of behavioral symptoms of dementia in the Introduction).

The neuropathology of anxiety in people with dementia is not well understood, as indicated by this: "It is difficult to determine whether the behavior is the result of neurodegeneration, cognitive dysfunction, previous experiences, current stressors, independently coexisting psychopathology, or a combination of these factors" (Bolger et al., 1994, p. 331).

For people with dementia, untreated anxiety results in unpleasant symptoms. Particularly in the early stages of dementia, episodes of uncharacteristic irritability or sensory misperceptions may alarm and frighten and provoke anxiety in people with dementia. They may experience a sense of fear about an upcoming event (Godot syndrome) and therefore ask repeated questions about it; or they may experience excessive fear of being left alone and, as a result, shadow the caregiver. Anxiety also may be evoked by suspiciousness, paranoia, delusions, or hallucinations (Bolger et al., 1994; Bungener, Jouvent, & Derouesne, 1996).

Mrs. Gloria Gomez, age 78, was admitted 1 week ago to a long-term care facility. She was diagnosed as having dementia 2 years ago, and had been living with her extended family until her need for care became greater than they could provide. At this time, additional medical diagnoses included chronic obstructive pulmonary disease (COPD) and osteoarthritis in her knees. Her son, Guillermo, and daughter-in-law, Gabriela, along with their children and Mrs. Gomez's sister, Gertrudes Goya, remain actively involved in her care. Mrs. Gomez has settled into the routine of the nursing facility, but she seems fretful. The nursing staff observe that her hands shake, her voice quivers, she becomes jittery when anyone except her family members touches her, and she cries, "I'm scared!" when she is led into the bathroom.

## ETIOLOGIES AND OUTCOMES OF ANXIETY

Anxiety can be a primary disorder, but more commonly it is a symptom of an illness or a response to stress. The etiologies and outcomes of anxiety are complex (Figure 7.1). As with all behavioral symptoms, a careful assessment of the person should be conducted to identify the cause so that interventions can be directed to the source of the problem.

> During Mrs. Gomez's initial assessment at the nursing facility, the social worker and nurse report that she has no history of an anxiety disorder. Guillermo, however, says that his mother became fretful when unfamiliar people visited them in their home. He also reported that when he and Gabriela tried to make his mother happy by telling her about an upcoming event, such as a birthday party for one of her grandchildren, she would rush around cleaning the house and asking them repeatedly when the people were coming. Not wanting to upset her, they decide not to tell her ahead of time about the move to the nursing facility.

### PRIMARY ANXIETY DISORDERS

The *Diagnostic and Statistical Manual of Mental Disorders, Fourth Edition* (American Psychiatric Association, 1994) includes a number of primary anxiety disorders, such as generalized anxiety disorder, phobias, post-traumatic stress disorder, and obsessive-compulsive disorders. The relevance of this diagnostic system for older adults, particularly those with dementia, has been questioned (McCarthy, Katz, & Foa, 1991; Yesavage & Taylor, 1991), therefore it may be more instructive to look at symptom patterns.

Individual symptoms of anxiety appear more frequently than does an anxiety disorder. This is true for older adults in general, and especially for people with dementia. In fact, new-onset primary anxiety disorders are unusual in older adults. In most instances, older people with primary anxiety disorders have a history of them, and it is therefore important to obtain a complete personal and family psychiatric history.

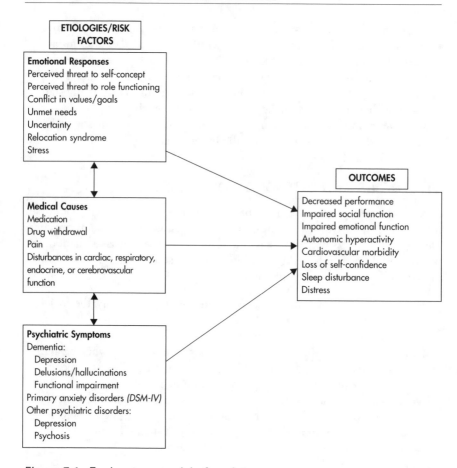

*Figure 7.1. Explanatory model of anxiety.*

## ANXIETY AS A SYMPTOM OF ILLNESS

Anxiety may be the symptom that marks the initial presentation of disease. New-onset anxiety usually is the result of a medical cause or a medication side effect. This emphasizes the need for a comprehensive medical and psychiatric evaluation prior to instituting treatment. Some medical conditions and medications that can produce symptoms of anxiety are listed in Table 7.1. The most common psychiatric disorder causing anxiety in later life is depression (Sussman, 1988).

Mrs. Gomez receives a bronchodilator via inhalation every 4 hours, and has an order for 2 liters of oxygen by nasal cannula as needed (PRN). About an hour before her scheduled treatment, she starts calling for a

**Table 7.1.   Medical conditions and medications that can produce symptoms of anxiety**

| Condition / process | Examples |
| --- | --- |
| Decreased oxygen to the brain | Cardiovascular disease: arrhythmias, congestive heart failure, hypotension<br>Pulmonary disease: asthma, chronic obstructive pulmonary disease, pulmonary emboli, respiratory infection |
| Endocrine | Hyperthyroidism<br>Hypoglycemia |
| Medication side effects | Anticholinergic drugs<br>Caffeine<br>Steroids<br>Sympathomimetics—decongestants/ bronchodilators<br>Alcohol<br>Narcotics<br>Sedative-hypnotics<br>Psychotropic medications |
| Withdrawal symptoms | Alcohol<br>Benzodiazepines (especially short acting)<br>Central nervous system depressants |

Data from Miller (1999) and Shamoian (1991).

nurse in a loud, panicky voice. When the nursing assistant responds, Mrs. Gomez pushes her away and screams, "Nurse!" louder. When the nurse arrives, Mrs. Gomez grabs her arm, shaking it back and forth, panting, "I can't breathe! I can't breathe!" The nurse checks Mrs. Gomez's oxygen saturation with the pulse oximeter and finds it to be an unsatisfactory 89%. Portable oxygen is set up and the nurse stays with Mrs. Gomez, holding her hands, speaking in a gentle voice, and modeling slow inspiration and pursed-lip expiration. After 5 minutes, Mrs. Gomez's oxygen saturation returns to 95% and she appears calm.

## ANXIETY AS A STRESS RESPONSE

Anxiety is a normal response to real or perceived threats to any of the following: health, assets, values, environment, self-concept, role function, needs fulfillment, goal achievement, personal relationships, and sense of security. In addition, anxiety also can arise from subconscious conflicts, maturational crises, developmental challenges, or fears of becoming a victim of crime or elder abuse. These sources of anxiety apply to any older person, including those who have dementia.

Older adults with dementia may be vulnerable to anxiety because the cognitive and physical impairments of dementia increase the frequency with which stressful losses occur and because the impairments interfere with previously effective coping mechanisms for dealing with stress. Specific environmental or situational factors also may contribute to anxiety. Expecting too much (or too little) of people with dementia or changing routines can lead to anxiety. In addition, anxiety in people with dementia may be a reflection of the caregiver's stress because people with dementia tend to mirror the emotions of those around them (Bolger et al., 1994; Stehman, Strachan, Glenner, Glenner, & Neubauer, 1996).

The progressively lowered stress threshold (PLST) model emphasizes the effect of the environment on people with dementia (Hall & Buckwalter, 1987). The PLST model postulates the increasing inability of people with dementia to cope with stress because of progressive cerebral pathology and associated cognitive decline. Both environmental and internal stressors create demands that can cause a person with dementia to become anxious. If the stressful stimuli continue, then behavior becomes increasingly dysfunctional and can lead to a catastrophic reaction (Gerdner, Hall, & Buckwalter, 1996).

## ASSESSMENT OF ANXIETY

A person with anxiety may verbalize feelings of apprehension, uncertainty, fear, distress, helplessness, inadequacy, or regret (Gordon, 1997). As the dementia progresses, the person's ability to verbalize such feelings is affected by cognitive and language deficits. Behavioral manifestations of anxiety may be present during any stage of dementia, but they become increasingly important in making the diagnosis of anxiety when verbalization of feelings is impaired.

It is important to assess whether the anxiety is situational or is the result of a more generalized anxiety disorder. In addition, knowing the severity of and response to previous stressors can help evaluate the person's ability to cope with current concerns and feelings (Bolger et al., 1994; Cohen-Mansfield, Marx, & Werner, 1992). The environment must be assessed for sources of anxiety (see Figure 7.1).

> Mrs. Gomez has many sources of anxiety (e.g., relocation to a new environment, strange caregivers, a new routine, some loss of independence, visual hallucinations, hypoxia). A comprehensive, person-centered plan of care is instituted to address each etiology.

Many common symptoms that are clinical indictors of anxiety have been identified (Table 7.2; because there is no accepted organizing theme, individual indicators are listed in the table). Several of these indicators also may be symp-

**Table 7.2.  Clinical indicators of anxiety**

| | | |
|---|---|---|
| Angry outbursts | Increased muscle tension | Scared |
| Asking repeated questions | Insomnia | Shadowing the caregiver |
| Changes in eating patterns | Irritability | Shakiness |
| Crying | Losing control | Tachycardia |
| Diaphoresis | Pacing | Tearfulness |
| Dry mouth | Poor attention span | Trembling |
| Facial tension | Poor eye contact | Urinary frequency |
| Fidgeting | Rapid, disconnected speech | Voice changes |
| Glancing about | Rattled | Voice quivering |
| Hyperventilation | Repetitive motions | Wariness |
| Inability to sit still | Restlessness | |

Data from Eliopoulus (1999), Gordon (1997), and Miller (1999).

toms of other conditions (e.g., "dry mouth" may be a symptom of anticholinergic medications, "changes in eating patterns" may be a symptom of acute illness). In any individual's care plan it is best to list the specific clinical indicators that lead to the conclusion of "anxiety." For example, a nurse's notes may read, "Anxiety, as indicated by trembling, rapid speech and shadowing of the caregiver."

The following questions and observations are suggested to assess anxiety in any setting:

• What are the clinical indicators of anxiety?
• What real or perceived threats are present that may be sources of anxiety for the person?
• Might caffeine, pathological conditions, medications, or unmet needs (e.g., hunger, pain, need to urinate) be contributing to the person's anxiety?
• How often do the person's symptoms of anxiety occur?
• What is the effect of anxiety on the person's daily life (e.g., performance, quality)?
• What coping mechanisms has the caregiver tried with the care recipient and what were their effects?

Ask the following questions of the person with dementia or of caregivers if the person is unable to respond because of cognitive or language impairments:

• "What kinds of things do you worry about?"
• "Do you ever have trouble with your nerves?"

## THERAPEUTIC GOALS AND INTERVENTIONS

In treating the anxious person with dementia, three important facts must be kept in mind. First, anxiety always is a response to real or perceived threats, even if the source of anxiety is not readily identified. Second, anxiety is distressing to the person who is experiencing it. Third, anxiety decreases performance. Treatment of anxiety can be directed toward management of the symptom or toward removing or minimizing its sources. A person-centered approach, in which the caregiver views the world from the perspective of the person with anxiety, is essential.

### ENVIRONMENT-FOCUSED INTERVENTIONS

Environmental stressors are common causes of anxiety. Therefore, interventions that eliminate or minimize these stressors may prevent anxiety. Researchers have shown that new experiences—for example, changes in environment or disruption of usual routines—are the most likely to elicit a stress response (Frazer, Molinoff, & Winokur, 1994; Preville et al., 1996). As a result of short-term memory loss, every day is a new and potentially stressful experience for the person with dementia. However, procedural memory is retained longer than the ability to form new memories. Therefore, rituals and consistency help to prevent anxiety. Sensitizing caregivers is an important strategy for reducing anxiety. For example, it is helpful for the caregiver to know that it is best to approach the person calmly from the front, to provide reassurance, to smile, to model calm behavior, and to not argue (Burgener, Jirovec, Murrell, & Barton, 1992). The person's behavior response is used to measure the success of these interventions. Calm and functional behavior is the desired outcome. This goal can be reached by promoting minimal levels of stress, enhancing feelings of trust and safety, and promoting control.

### Minimizing Stress Level

The PLST model suggests that reducing stress by modifying environmental demands promotes adaptive behavior (Gerdner et al., 1996). Interventions that are based on principles from this model (Table 7.3) are designed to gear the environment to the person's level of function by minimizing the levels of stress—neither overstimulating nor understimulating. Although more research is needed, the model makes intuitive sense, and the interventions are good practices.

### Enhancing Feelings of Trust and Safety

Safety and security are basic human needs. The person with dementia needs to be safe and to feel safe. People with impaired cognitive function are still

**Table 7.3. Interventions that minimize stress levels**

| Principle of PLST model | Intervention |
|---|---|
| 1. Maximize the level of safe function | Promote rest periods to prevent fatigue and reduce stress.<br>Support all areas of loss in a prosthetic manner (e.g., be the person's "crutch" without decreasing his or her independence). |
| 2. Provide unconditional positive regard | Address person distinctly by name when initiating interaction and speak slowly.<br>Introduce self when making contact.<br>Speak in a clear, low, warm, respectful tone of voice.<br>Prepare for interaction with eye contact and touch as appropriate.<br>Avoid the use of physical restraints. |
| 3. Assess behavioral indicators of anxiety to determine appropriate levels of activity and stimuli | Determine behavioral expectations appropriate to the person's cognitive status.<br>Avoid frustrating the person by quizzing him or her with orientation questions that cannot be answered.<br>Ask family and friends to see the person only singly or a pair at a time to prevent overstimulation.<br>Limit choices to a number that does not cause the person anxiety.<br>Give one simple direction at a time.<br>Avoid touch and close proximity if they cause stress.<br>Use distraction rather than confrontation to manage behavior. |
| 4. Teach caregivers to "listen" to the person by evaluating verbal and nonverbal responses | Identify usual patterns of behavior for such activities as sleep, medication use, elimination, food intake, and self-care.<br>Use change in usual pattern as an indicator of stress. |
| 5. Modify the environments to support losses and enhance safety | Provide a low-stimulation environment (e.g., soothing music; nonvivid and simple, familiar patterns in decor; performance expectations that do not exceed cognitive processing ability; dining in small groups).<br>Decrease noise levels by avoiding paging systems and call lights that ring or buzz.<br>To promote orientation, provide cues such as current events, seasons, location, and names.<br>Remove or cover mirrors if the person is frightened by them.<br>Provide caregivers that are familiar to the person.<br>Avoid unfamiliar situations when possible.<br>Provide adequate, nonglare lighting.<br>Select activities based on cognitive processing abilities and interests. |
| 6. Provide ongoing education, support, care, and problem solving for caregivers | Determine the person's physical, social, and psychological history, usual habits, routines, and coping strategies.<br>Discuss with family members and friends how best to interact with the person. |

From Gerdner, L.A., Hall, G.R., & Buckwalter, K.C. (1996). Caregiver training for people with Alzheimer's based on a stress threshold model. *Image: The Journal of Nursing Scholarship, 28*, 241–246.

117

sensitive to others' attitudes, and they can respond to both caregiver stress and caregiver calmness.

> Mrs. Gomez exhibits so much anxiety between the time she is told she is going to take a bath and the time she is taken to the tub room that the nursing staff decide to give her a towel bath in bed. They also try to minimize her negative anticipation by gently explaining what they are about to do (e.g., "I'm going to wash your face now"). This approach is effective in decreasing Mrs. Gomez's anxiety, until she is turned onto her side, when she again begins to tremble and cry. The siderail, which Mrs. Gomez is facing, is lifted so she can hold onto it while her back is being washed. The nursing assistant quickly remembers that "being safe" and "feeling safe" are not the same concept. Thus, while Mrs. Gomez is having her back washed, a second caregiver makes eye contact with her, smiles, and talks gently to her. Mrs. Gomez's sister, Gertrudes, often comes to visit at bathtime and plays this role. Gertrudes loves participating in her sister's care in a meaningful way. Mrs. Gomez smiles and seems engaged in their conversations, even though she does not understand the words.

## Promoting Control

Promoting control should prevent anxiety that is caused by perceived threats to a person's independence, self-esteem, or role function (see Chapter 5).

### BEHAVIORAL INTERVENTIONS

Cognitive-behavioral therapies, such as progressive relaxation and sensory imagery, are effective for mild forms of anxiety (Rothschild & Rothschild, 1998). These therapies can be adapted for people with dementia across all levels of the disease.

## Music Therapy

The capacity to perceive and enjoy music usually is preserved in people with dementia (see Chapter 6). Music reduces their stress level, strengthens their immune systems, and acts as a catalyst to improve their human interactions (Ragneskog, Kihlgren, Karlsson, & Norberg, 1996). Researchers have found that classical music, soothing nature sounds, or favorite music played during activities of daily living, such as recreation therapy and preparation for bedtime, is effective in decreasing anxiety and promoting relaxation (Casby & Holm, 1994; Gerdner, 1997; Ragneskog et al., 1996). Whatever works should be used.

> Mrs. Gomez loves church hymns and the songs she used to sing to her

grandchildren. Her family brings a tape recording of the church choir's Christmas concert, and the grandchildren make a tape of songs they remember singing with their grandmother. The recreation therapy department finds a tape with Lawrence Welk and Mitch Miller sing-alongs. Nursing staff keep a log, recording the reasons they turn on the tape and Mrs. Gomez's responses. They find that if they turn on the tape when Mrs. Gomez shows the first signs of anxiety, she will gently rock, sometimes hum along, and occasionally join in for a phrase or two.

## Reminiscence

Many people with dementia live in the past, and remembering fond events can be very pleasurable. Reminiscence, or the recall of past events, has been used successfully in people with dementia to bring pleasure to their lives (Kovach, 1991; Rentz, 1995; see also "Simulated Presence Therapy" in Chapters 6 and 12).

Gertrudes visits often. On several occasions, the staff observe the sisters' animated conversations about their past—how Mrs. Gomez met her husband on a train; the day they picked apples from a neighbor's tree and almost got caught; the glorious wedding cake they baked together that would not rise; their childhood dog Paco; the day that Gloria was picked May Queen. Gertrudes sings to Mrs. Gomez in their native Spanish and brings her sister's favorite foods. Together, they look through old photo albums. These are the best times. Mrs. Gomez is animated and smiling and seems happy and engaged. The staff write down these memories and use them as topics of conversation during care.

## Snoezelen

Snoezelen is a recreational therapy and diversion program that is designed to relax people (see Chapter 6). The program includes music combined with light that is shone through colored oils to project moving images of colored bubbles onto a screen or wall. For example, with blue hues, relaxing music is played. Snoezelen's broad objective is to provide an interesting and relaxing atmosphere by invoking the use of the senses. Snoezelen has been used with older adults to promote relaxation and to decrease resistiveness during dental care (Volicer, Mahoney, & Brown, 1998).

## PHARMACOLOGICAL INTERVENTIONS

Nonpharmacological behavioral interventions should always be considered the first approach to treatment. Medications often are used as a default means of patient care management, despite the known disadvantages (Weinrich,

Egbert, Eleazer, & Haddock, 1995). In fact, the Nursing Home Reform Act, which was included in the Omnibus Budget Reconciliation Act of 1987, specifically mandates against the use of "chemical restraints imposed for purposes of discipline or convenience and not required to treat the resident's medical symptoms" (Omnibus Budget Reconciliation Act, 1987, p. 1330-165). Therefore, it is important to assess specific symptoms, weigh risks and benefits, and identify instances when medication will improve the quality of life for the person who has anxiety. One criterion for medication use states, "If behavioral measures fail or the anxiety is so severe that it threatens to destabilize the person's medical status, medication should be used" (Sussman, 1988, p. 4).

Caution must be used when prescribing drugs that might interfere with remaining cognitive function. Drug treatment alone is an insufficient therapy. In fact, because of the cognitive vulnerability of people with dementia, behavioral interventions actually may be preferable to psychopharmacological treatment (Bolger et al., 1994).

The most commonly prescribed medications are short-acting anxiolytic drugs from the benzodiazepine class of sedative-hypnotics, and buspirone. The anxiolytic effects of benzodiazepines result from depressing neurotransmission in the limbic system and cortical areas. Guidelines for the initiation of anxiolytics are listed in Table 7.4, and examples of their most common side effects are given in Table 7.5. When anxiolytics are prescribed for symptom management, the lowest possible dose should be used for the shortest possible time. When symptoms decrease, a drug holiday should be considered.

Mrs. Gomez requires excision of a broken tooth that is causing her pain and difficulty in eating. On a previous trip to the dental clinic, she became so anxious that the procedure had to be canceled even though she had been accompanied by her sister, the clinic was in the same building in which she lives, and relaxing music was playing in the background of the dentist's office. To prevent another catastrophic reaction, the physician orders lorazepam, 0.5 mg, to be given 1 hour before the dental procedure. This one-time use is indicated to help Mrs. Gomez cope with the necessary procedure. She is at risk for respiratory depression, a lorazepam side effect, because of her COPD history. Her

**Table 7.4.    Guidelines for initiating anxiolytic medications**

Establish a clear-cut indication for their use.

Identify those patients most vulnerable to adverse effects.

Select a specific drug based on solid knowledge.

Monitor treatment continuously.

Use drugs with short to intermediate half-lives.

Prescribe small doses for brief periods.

Adapted from Salzman (1991) and Sussman (1988).

Table 7.5.  Selected medications to treat anxiety

| Drug class | Name (trade name) | Dose range and frequency[a] | Half-life (hours) | Side effects |
|---|---|---|---|---|
| Benzodiazepines | Lorazepam (Ativan) | 0.5–1 mg BID or TID | 15 | • Sedation<br>• Impaired motor coordination<br>• Akathisia<br>• Risk of falls<br>• Memory loss<br>• Respiratory depression<br>• Central nervous system depression<br>• Withdrawal (taper off slowly)<br>• Paradoxical reaction |
|  | Alprazolam (Xanax) | 0.25–0.5 mg TID | 12 | |
|  | Oxazepam (Serax) | 10–20 mg TID or QID | 8 | |
|  | Clonazepam (Klonopin) | 0.25–0.5 mg BID | 34 | |
| Azapirones | Buspirone (Buspar) | 5–20 mg TID | (onset of action 3–6 weeks) | Headache<br>Nausea<br>Drowsiness<br>Lightheadedness |
| Antidepressants | (see Chapter 3) | | | |
| Antipsychotics | (see Chapter 4) | | | |

Data from Raskind (1998) and Stone et al. (1999).

respiratory status is stable, however, and a low dose is prescribed. She is monitored for any change in her status. The side effect of sedation is beneficial in this time-limited situation. There is no functional impairment because the short half-life of lorazepam means that the medication effects will not linger beyond their clinical indication.

Gertrudes accompanies Mrs. Gomez to the dental clinic again, this time singing along the way. The dentist plays music from a tape of Mrs. Gomez's favorite songs. The tooth extraction is completed, and Mrs. Gomez remains calm throughout the procedure. Two hours after returning to the nursing unit, Mrs. Gomez begins to cry. Her body language is tense and she is fidgeting with rather than eating her dinner. The nurse assesses these as signs of discomfort and administers an analgesic. Mrs. Gomez only eats half of her dinner, but she sleeps well during the night. The next day she is back to her usual self.

If anxiety is a symptom of depression, then an antidepressant will alleviate it (Rothschild & Rothschild, 1998). If hallucinations precipitate anxiety, as in the case of Mrs. Gomez, then antipsychotics may effectively prevent it by treating the cause.

> Mrs. Gomez seems anxious. When she is alone, she cries quietly and fidgets with the bedclothes. She rocks a baby doll in her arms. When the nurse enters her room and turns toward the bathroom, Mrs. Gomez starts screaming, "No, no, don't go there! Please help me!" Mrs. Gomez becomes diaphoretic and her pulse rises dramatically to 110 beats per minute. The nurse knows that Mrs. Gomez has an order for PRN lorazepam, but before giving the medication, she tries to comfort Mrs. Gomez. When the nurse enters the bathroom to retrieve a cool wash-cloth for Mrs. Gomez's face, Mrs. Gomez again screams, "Don't go there! Don't you see the smoke? Fire! Fire! The bathroom's on fire! Help! Help!" The nurse quickly returns to Mrs. Gomez's side. In an attempt to distract her, the nurse comments on how pretty the baby doll is. Mrs. Gomez again starts screaming and pulls the doll away from the nurse's outreached hand. "Don't touch her! Can't you see she has no head?" Mrs. Gomez is started on risperidone 0.25 mg daily to prevent her hal-lucinations. Within a week, she no longer experiences these terrifying hallucinations. As a result, her symptoms of anxiety also decrease markedly, to the point at which she is able to respond to music and Snoezelen. These therapies are started at least 30 minutes before initiat-ing activities that Mrs. Gomez finds stressful.

## REFERENCES

American Psychiatric Association. (1994). *Diagnostic and statistical manual of mental disorders* (4th ed.). Washington, DC: American Psychiatric Press.
Bolger, J.P., Carpenter, B.D., & Strauss, M.E. (1994). Behavior and affect in Alzheimer's disease. *Clinics in Geriatric Medicine, 10*(2), 315–337.
Bungener, C., Jouvent, R., & Derouesne, C. (1996). Affective disturbances in Alzheimer's disease. *Journal of the American Geriatrics Society, 44*, 1066–1071.
Burgener, S.C., Jirovec, M., Murrell, L., & Barton, D. (1992). Caregiver and environ-mental variables related to difficult behaviors in institutionalized demented elderly persons. *Journal of Gerontology: Psychological Sciences, 47*, P242–P249.
Casby, J.A., & Holm, M.B. (1994). The effect of music on repetitive disruptive vocal-izations of persons with dementia. *American Journal of Occupational Therapy, 48*, 883–889.
Cohen-Mansfield, J., Marx, M.S., & Werner, P. (1992). Agitation in elderly persons: An integrative report of findings in a nursing home. *International Psychogeriatrics, 4*, 221–240.
Eliopoulos, C. (1999). *Manual of gerontologic nursing.* St. Louis: Mosby.
Folks, D.G. (1999). Management of anxiety in the long-term care setting. *Annals of Long-Term Care, 7*(2), 44–50.

Frazer, A., Molinoff, P.B., & Winokur, A. (Eds.) (1994). *Biological bases of brain function and disease.* New York: Raven Press.

Gerdner, L. (1997). An individualized music intervention for agitation. *Journal of the American Psychiatric Nurses Association, 3,* 177–184.

Gerdner, L.A., Hall, G.R., & Buckwalter, K.C. (1996). Caregiver training for people with Alzheimer's based on a stress threshold model. *Image: The Journal of Nursing Scholarship, 28,* 241–246.

Gordon, M. (1997). *Manual of nursing diagnosis 1997–1998.* St. Louis: Mosby.

Hall, G.R., & Buckwalter, K.C. (1987). Progressively lowered stress threshold: A conceptual model for care of adults with Alzheimer's disease. *Archives of Psychiatric Nursing, 1,* 399–406.

Jost, B.C., & Grossberg, G.T. (1996). The evolution of psychiatric symptoms in Alzheimer's disease: A natural history study. *Journal of the American Geriatrics Society, 44,* 1978–1981.

Kovach, C.R. (1991). Reminiscence behavior: An empirical exploration. *Journal of Gerontological Nursing, 17*(12), 23–28.

Logsdon, R.G., & Teri, L. (1997). The Pleasant Events Schedule-AD: Psychometric properties and relationship to depression and cognition in Alzheimer's disease patients. *Gerontologist, 37,* 40–45.

McCarthy, P.R., Katz, I.R., & Foa, E.B. (1991). Cognitive-behavioral treatment of anxiety in the elderly: A proposed model. In C. Salzman & B.D. Lebowitz (Eds.), *Anxiety in the elderly* (pp. 197–214). New York: Springer.

Miller, C.A. (1999). *Nursing care of older adults* (3rd ed.). Philadelphia: Lippincott.

Omnibus Budget Reconciliation Act of 1987, PL 101-203, 42 C.F.R. § 483 *et seq.*

Preville, M., Susman, E., Zarit, S.H., Smyer, M., Bosworth, H.G., & Reid, J.D. (1996). A measurement model of cortisol reactivity of healthy older adults. *Journal of Gerontology: Psychological Sciences, 51B,* P64–P69.

Ragneskog, H., Kihlgren, M., Karlsson, I., & Norberg, A. (1996). Dinner music for demented patients. *Clinical Nursing Research, 5,* 262–282.

Raskind, M.A. (1998). Psychopharmacology of noncognitive abnormal behaviors in Alzheimer's disease. *Journal of Clinical Psychiatry, 59*(Suppl. 9), 28–32.

Rentz, C.A. (1995). Reminiscence: A supportive intervention for the person with Alzheimer's disease. *Journal of Psychosocial Nursing, 33*(11), 15–20.

Rothschild, J.A., & Rothschild, A.J. (1998). Psychotropics in primary care. In L.A. Eisenhauer & M.A. Murphy (Eds.), *Pharmacotherapeutics and advanced nursing practice* (pp. 337–374). New York: McGraw-Hill.

Salzman, C. (1991). Pharmacologic treatment of the anxious elderly patient. In C. Salzman & B.D. Lebowitz (Eds.), *Anxiety in the elderly* (pp. 149–173). New York: Springer.

Shamoian, C.A. (1991). What is anxiety in the elderly? In C. Salzman & B.D. Lebowitz (Eds.), *Anxiety in the elderly* (pp. 3–15). New York: Springer.

Stehman, J.M., Strachan, G.I., Glenner, J.A., Glenner, G.G., & Neubauer, J.K. (1996). *Handbook of dementia care.* Baltimore: The Johns Hopkins University Press.

Stone, J.T., Wyman, J.F., & Salisbury, S.A. (1999). *Clinical gerontological nursing: A guide to advanced practice* (2nd ed.). Philadelphia: W.B. Saunders.

Sussman, N. (1988). Diagnosis and drug treatment of anxiety in the elderly. *Geriatric Medicine Today, 7*(10), 1–8.

Volicer, L., Mahoney, E., & Brown, E.J. (1998). Nonpharmacological approaches to the management of the behavioral consequences of advanced dementia. In M. Kaplan & S.B. Hoffman (Eds.), *Behaviors in dementia: Best practices for successful management* (pp. 155–176). Baltimore: Health Professions Press.

Weinrich, S., Egbert, C., Eleazer, D.P., & Haddock, K.S. (1995). Agitation: Measurement, management, and intervention research. *Archives of Psychiatric Nursing, 9,* 251–260.

Yesavage, J.A., & Taylor, B. (1991). Anxiety and dementia. In C. Salzman & B.D. Lebowitz (Eds.), *Anxiety in the elderly* (pp. 79–85). New York: Springer.

# 8

# Spatial Disorientation

Spatial disorientation means misperceiving immediate surroundings, not being aware of one's setting, or not knowing where one is in relation to the environment. Even when a person can see clearly, space and location may be distorted, objects may be interpreted incorrectly, or directions may be misunderstood. Spatial disorientation may cause misunderstanding of the environment and lead to the development of fear, anxiety, suspicions, illusions, delusions, and safety problems such as getting lost. In the early stages of dementia, the person with the disease may become confused when in an unfamiliar place. In the later stages the person can become confused when in previously familiar places.

Harry Henley is a 66-year-old man who was diagnosed as having dementia a year ago, just after he retired from his position as chief executive officer of a Fortune 500 technology firm. He lives with his wife Helen in a large house with an in-ground pool and tennis court. It is located in an affluent suburb of a large east coast city, three blocks from their country club. Harry spent many years climbing the corporate ladder. He thought that helping out at home was not manly and was beneath him. He loved golf, and he served on some very large corporations' boards of directors. Now, Harry, who used to be the "in-charge" person, cannot manage his own spending money. He would not be well dressed if Helen did not select his wardrobe and place his clothing for the day in his dressing room. Helen makes sure he has cash in his wallet, and reminds him of his golf dates. An hour after Helen waves goodbye to Harry in the driveway as he leaves for the club, she receives a call from one of Harry's golfing partners inquiring into Harry's whereabouts.

Instead of driving the same three blocks to the country club that he has driven for 20 years, Harry, who never shops, drives to the local farm stand, parks the car, and wanders about politely nodding hello to people. He is lost. The farm stand is not his "territory." The next call that Helen receives is from the farm stand owner, who recognizes one of the Henley's cars. Helen drives there and finds her husband standing next to his car, watching people come and go.

## WALKING THE WALK OF THE DISORIENTED PERSON WITH DEMENTIA

Successfully managing the challenging behavior of a person with dementia requires more than "book knowledge." It requires the humane, empathetic, and skillful application of evidence-based interventions. This is especially important for helping people who are disoriented. One way of promoting skill application is to understand what it is like for the person with spatial disorientation problems. Applying personal experiences to the situation of another (e.g., dealing with pain, coping with fear of the dentist, living with the flu) can help convey an emotional understanding from the caregiver to the care recipient. If a caregiver, such as a certified nursing assistant (CNA), has not experienced some of the problems experienced by care recipients, then the caregiver can learn experientially in a classroom setting. For instance, to help a person with right-sided hemiplegia resulting from a stroke, a class of CNAs can be given the exercise of changing from one set of clothing to another without using their right arms or legs. Another assignment to improve the care of people with visual impairment can be to again change a set of clothing, but do it while blindfolded.

There is no exercise to teach caregivers how to provide empathetic care to the person with dementia and spatial disorientation by experiencing a similar situation, but several analogies have been proposed. One analogy is the "Wizard of Alz," an experience developed by Barbara Helm (director of The Breckinridge, Lexington, Kentucky), based on *The Wizard of Oz*. Here, one mentally walks with Dorothy, the girl from Kansas who, with her dog, Toto, struggles to find the Emerald City after she wakes up in the Land of Oz. All of the people in Oz looked very different from Dorothy (e.g., the munchkins were very small), and someone (the Wicked Witch of the West) was out to get her. Dorothy was driven by her need to go home to Kansas and was told she could get home by consulting the Wizard of Oz in the Emerald City. During her journey to the Emerald City, Dorothy faced many obstacles. She was frightened by apple trees throwing apples at her and by meeting the Lion, the Scarecrow, and the Tin Man, who had familiar human characteristics. Dorothy also became intoxicated in a poppy field, was terrorized by flying monkeys, and encountered unmarked road signs pointing in different directions.

Harry Henley was lost in very familiar territory. Instead of driving the same few blocks he drove so often, he went in another direction and ended up in a parking lot, but not the intended one. Luckily for Harry, he did not drive for miles and end up where neither he nor his car would be recognized. Some other people with dementia are not so lucky, and they become missing persons (see Chapter 13). People with mild dementia usually are oriented to their environment when they are in familiar surroundings. They may get confused, however, if they become stressed or if they are moved to a new location, such as adult day services or a vacation spot. When there are no interpretable signs or familiar cues, or if familiar objects, routes, or signs are misinterpreted, the person can get lost, feel uncomfortable, and become frightened.

## RATIONALE FOR INTERVENTIONS TO MANAGE SPATIAL DISORIENTATION

Spatial disorientation, a secondary symptom of dementia, is a very general condition, but it is a consequence of specific pathological changes that occur in several areas of the brain. Understanding the etiologies of spatial disorientation allows caregivers to plan interventions that may compensate for its specific pathology.

### PATHOPHYSIOLOGICAL CAUSES

The pathological processes of dementing illnesses cause problems in spatial orientation by directly damaging the posterior cingulate gyrus and hippocampus. The posterior cingulate gyrus is one of the cerebral hemisphere convolutions. In a study of 86 people with mild to moderate Alzheimer's disease, hypofunction of the posterior cingulate gyrus, identified through positron emission tomography (PET) scan measurement of glucose metabolism, was found to be associated with disorientation for place (Hirono et al., 1998). The hippocampus is a memory structure located in the temporal lobes of the brain that is associated with spatial memory. The hippocampus is necessary for place navigation in both humans and nonhuman animals (Holden & Therrien, 1989). An individual with a healthy hippocampus uses two mechanisms to find his or her way: cognitive mapping and cue navigation. *Cognitive mapping* requires cognitive processing to identify and store mental images of the most frequently encountered elements in a particular environment and the ability to make the connections among those elements. Objects in an environment and their spatial contexts are stored in memory as mental images or patterns that are generated after repeated contact with the environment. This way, people can navigate in their environment and "see" not only the route but also alternate routes.

The second mechanism for wayfinding is *cue navigation,* a process that works by the selection and use of a single landmark (cue) that directs an individual toward a specific location within the environment. When hippocampal damage occurs, single-cue navigation is possible if the posterior parietal lobe is functional. For cue navigation to be effective, the individual must have the capacity to remember the cue and its role in that environment. Individuals retain those cues longer when they are familiar and are strongly associated with an environmental landmark (Holden & Therrien, 1993).

The pathological processes of dementing illness indirectly cause problems through impairment in visual attention, dysfunction in depth perception, and visual agnosia. In addition to the primary memory deficit of dementia, another problem is attentional impairment, that is, not being able to stay focused or to concentrate on a task. The ability to initiate or sustain visual focus is an aspect of selective visual attention that allows a person to attend to a particular region of extrapersonal space and rapidly obtain accurate information about that location. Because of pathology in the specific area of the brain that contributes to spatial orientation, individuals with dementia have deficits in shifting their visual attention from an incorrectly cued location to another location, changing attention between different features of a cue, shifting between visual and auditory modalities, and moving from one stimulus set or categorization rule to another. For example, Harry Henley was not where he wanted to be, and he did not have the capacity to self-correct the situation. Harry had difficulty shifting his attention from his car to the parking lot; or, when looking at the parking lot, to change from focusing on its ground color to its size; or to shift between looking at the parking lot and listening to the farm stand owner speaking to him.

Depth perception is a basic visual function that provides the ability to recognize that an object has depth as well as height and width, that is, that the object is three-dimensional. When compared with people without dementia, people with Alzheimer's disease were found to have significant impairments in both binocular and monocular depth perception (Mendez, Cherrier, & Meadows, 1996). Impaired depth perception causes visuospatial deficits and contributes to difficulties that people with dementia experience with navigating their environments, driving an automobile, orienting themselves in space, or recognizing visual objects. To Mr. Henley, a gully at the edge of the parking lot could look like a dark mark on the gravel surface or a dark shadow could look like a huge black hole.

Visual agnosia is a deficit in which people appear to use information about selected parts of an object in isolation from the object as a whole. The person may identify a particular element of a complex object or picture and be able to select a second element, but he or she may not be able to integrate the elements to correctly identify the object. Visual agnosia is similar to using the zoom lens on a camera to focus on one specific feature rather than using a panoramic lens to capture the total picture. Mr. Henley was in the wrong parking lot and, instead of "seeing" the entire farm stand parking lot, he saw only his own car.

## BASIS FOR INTERVENTIONS

Environmental interventions that are based on what the person with dementia sees are the cornerstone of management strategies for spatial disorientation. Research in two areas provides the theoretical basis for interventions: using cue familiarity to promote wayfinding by accommodating spatial disorientation following hippocampal damage (Holden & Therrien, 1993) and enhancing environmental cues during visual search to adjust for impaired visual attention (Greenwood, Parasuraman, & Alexander, 1997). For environmental cues to be effective in managing spatial disorientation, the relationship between the cue and the desired location must be maintained and the individual must be able to readily see the cue. Application of this research to clinical practice has identified two basic concepts that clinicians can use to create individualized strategies for people with dementia and spatial disorientation: pop-up cues and environmental landmarks.

*Pop-up cues* provide the rationale for color contrasts. When an individual without dementia looks at an object, he or she uses a combination of basic features (e.g., color, size, orientation, motion) and serially examines each feature to identify the object. Carrying out these steps requires repeated deployment of one's visuospatial attention across the visual field. The individual without dementia uses the recollection of these accumulated data to process and identify the object. In contrast, another approach that does not require using accumulated data is to use targets that differ from distractions by one single salient feature, which produces the phenomenon of pop-up. Looking for a pop-up does not require people to shift their visuospatial attention across features, to identify more than one salient feature of the object, or to remember features of the object. Using the pop-up cue can help when an individual with dementia does not use a white toilet in a white bathroom or will not sit on a blue chair in front of a blue wall. Specific color-cued interventions should be targeted to individuals in their environment (e.g., paint the bathroom wall red to provide color contrast to the white toilet, put a red chair in front of the blue wall).

*Environmental landmarks* should capitalize on long-standing memory and use objects that are associated with the years that the individual remembers best. In general, caregivers in the home environment should keep the same furniture in the same place, add no new furniture, and not change the decorations in rooms except to simplify the rooms and remove clutter. Clutter is a safety issue because the person with dementia will not understand what it is, may trip over it, and may become more confused because of it. Those personal effects that have long been associated with specific rooms or activities, however, should be used as orientation devices.

The behaviors of people with dementia have causes that seem logical to them, despite their inability to process cognitively. Spatial disorientation may stimulate people to enter or avoid specific areas. If a person will not go into a certain room, then there probably is a reason. For instance, if a large black shadow is in front of the entrance, the person with dementia may perceive that a black pool of water is preventing him or her from entering. Conversely, to prevent a person with dementia from leaving an area unaccompanied or from roaming into an unsafe or "off-limits" area, camouflage may be used to disguise the exit/entry.

## MODEL OF SPATIAL DISORIENTATION

The overall model of behavioral symptoms of dementia presented in the Introduction provides a conceptual framework for understanding relationships among the 13 challenging behaviors presented in this book. Figure 8.1 places spatial disorientation in the center of a model and illustrates relationships among the antecedents and effects of this behavioral symptom.

The dementing process, the central component of the overall conceptual framework, is presented in the upper right corner of Figure 8.1. The dementing process predisposes a person to spatial disorientation through symptoms of agnosia and inattention as well as deficits of depth perception, cue use, and cognitive mapping. A less-than-desirable environment, especially one with inappropriate lighting and shadows or a setting that is unfamiliar to the person with dementia, further exacerbates his or her spatial disorientation.

Delusions and hallucinations are core processes in the overall conceptual model and are both a direct antecedent and effect of spatial disorientation through the mechanisms of suspicion and fear. Suspicion and fear exacerbate or initiate a chain of events of increasing anxiety, which in turn can cause agitation, which leads to both worsening of deficits in activities of daily living (ADLs) and interference with other people. Spatial disorientation directly inhibits the ability of people with dementia to reach the place that they are

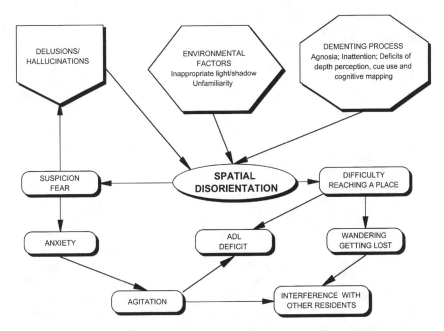

*Figure 8.1. Relationships between the antecedents and effects of spatial dis-orientation.*

seeking. Not reaching a desired place leads to further decrements in ADLs (e.g., when people cannot find the bathroom and become incontinent). People's unsuccessful attempts to reach a destination lead to wandering and becoming lost. People with dementia who are lost or wander through a residential facility into the rooms of other residents interfere with other residents.

There is no intervention to treat the underlying dementing process, but there are interventions to treat every other factor that can increase spatial disorientation. Effective interventions carried out by knowledgeable caregivers can decrease the negative consequences of spatial disorientation for people with dementia, other residents, and caregivers. If people with dementia live in a caregiving and structural environment that makes it easy and safe for them to move about and reach the appropriate destination, then wandering and becoming lost can be prevented. The caregivers' goal is to prevent the exacerbation of other problematic symptoms by planning and directing interventions to the underlying etiology by treating or compensating for specific pathological processes.

# MANAGEMENT SUGGESTIONS
# FOR SPATIAL DISORIENTATION

Every person is unique. Care plans should be individualized to the needs of each person, rather than to develop a boilerplate plan that is applied to all people. Strategies that are specific to the individual's degree of confusion and disorientation should be developed to allow independence while preventing injury and accidents.

Helen Henley was mortified to learn that she must collect her husband from the farm stand. Although the Henleys have no financial concerns and hire employees to assist them with running the household and land-scaping their property, Helen is very private about Harry's dementia. In an effort to shield Harry and herself from further embarrassing situa-tions, Helen decided that Harry should not go out alone anymore. Harry, however, is not accustomed to being told what he can and cannot do, and Helen's decision prompts many arguments about using the car. Helen tried to reason with Harry, but he no longer has the capacity to reason. Helen took all of the car keys and keeps them locked in her dresser drawer. Because Harry enjoyed walking many miles a week dur-ing his golf games, Helen decided that a good substitute for driving would be for him to walk in their yard. She had the swimming pool filled in and the entire yard fenced. Harry could exercise by walking in the yard, and she did not have to worry about him.

Some time later, two events alarmed Helen: Harry began voiding in the front hall coat closet. Then, one afternoon, Helen could not see Harry in the backyard. When she went outside to check on him, she found Harry standing in a corner of the yard. He had been following the fence, and, when it led to a right angle, he was unable to turn to the left. As a result, he stood there until he was "rescued."

## MILD DEMENTIA

Early in the dementing illness, while in a familiar environment and not stressed, the person with dementia should be able to walk to nearby places unescorted. In the mild stage, becoming lost is the most serious complication of spatial disorientation. People with dementia cannot self-correct or think their way out of a situation by visualizing the alternative route. When they become lost, they do not have the capacity to ask for directions, and they may not respond to hearing their names called. Staying in familiar environments is beneficial for the person with dementia. A caregiver may benefit from a vaca-tion with a change of scenery, but the combination of being in a different place and being removed from familiar surroundings may prompt more confusion and increase spatial disorientation for people with dementia.

Driving is one of the most difficult issues for an individual with dementia, and it should be resolved in this stage. Driving safely is affected by

- Cognitive symptoms of memory loss
- Inability to reason
- Poor judgment
- Functional problems of agnosia and apraxia
- Psychiatric symptoms of depression that may result in angry outbursts
- Unpleasant paranoid delusions or hallucinations
- Anxiety
- Agitation

The person with dementia experiences delayed reaction time and cannot recognize a safety hazard. Spatial disorientation leads to the development of fear, anxiety, suspicions, illusions, delusions, and loss of one's way. A person with these deficits should not drive. Driving is a risk for the person with dementia, and it may result in accidents and injury or death of the person or others. When the person should surrender the car keys is a difficult issue (Barr & Foley, 1993). The symptoms of dementia make driving a critical safety concern, and the caregiver must make the decision as to when the person with dementia can no longer drive (Odenheimer et al., 1994; Reinah, 1997).

## MODERATE DEMENTIA

In moderate dementia, intervention strategies should focus on dementia-appropriate environmental modifications and establishment of particular cues to preserve remaining independence. Just as one childproofs a home so that a toddler can be safe while developing walking and climbing skills, so should the environment for an individual with dementia be adjusted to allow for "sheltered freedom." Mrs. Henley should help Harry live in and navigate his environment. It is possible to teach environmental cues in the early stage of dementia before the hippocampal pathology is so extensive that no new learning can occur. The use of medications to enhance cognition (see Chapter 1) in the early stage of the disease suggests that more people will remain in the mild and moderate stages for a longer period of time. Thus, there is good reason to structure the environment by the placement of cues to direct behavior and wayfinding.

Mr. Henley is not incontinent. He must have recognized his need to void because he entered a small private room to do so, and he had the ability to walk independently and urinate without assistance. He simply mistook the closet for the bathroom. Harry has the physical ability to walk for miles every day in his large, enclosed backyard. Unfortunately, he gets stuck in corners.

If Mrs. Henley had requested professional assistance, then several modifications could have been put in place for Harry. For example, the following strategies would have helped Harry find the bathroom:

- Select one bathroom on each floor of the home for Harry to use.
- Paint the doors a light, bright color to contrast with the surrounding wall.
- Leave the doors partially ajar.
- Place a visual cue on the door (picture of a toilet) that Harry would associate with the bathroom.
- Keep small night-lights lit in the bathrooms.
- Place grab bars along the wall to guide the path to each bathroom.
- Light a visual path from the bedroom to the upstairs bathroom.
- Construct a visual path to the downstairs bathroom by visual cues (arrows pointing to it or pictures or other tactile cues to guide Harry to the bathroom door).
- Remove any obstacles (e.g., furniture, shadows, glare) from established bathroom paths.
- Paint the walls behind the toilets a bright color to contrast with white toilets.
- Cover the mirrors.
- Keep the interior simple by removing all extraneous objects and scatter rugs.

To prevent Mr. Henley from getting "stuck in the corner" in the yard, Helen could arrange for a number of alterations. She should consider the following options:

- Remove the fence angles and replace them with curves.
- Establish a level walking path.
- Avoid marks or dark spots in the light-colored path that could be misinterpreted as a hole or cliff.
- Light the area so that it is visible and does not cast shadows that can distort reality.
- Plant edible flowers and herbs to border the path and provide color contrast.
- Place a bench or chair nearby so that Harry can rest when he gets tired.

## SEVERE DEMENTIA

Four years after his diagnosis, Harry Henley's condition had markedly worsened. Despite being able to afford 24-hour assistance with personal care in their home, Helen could not bear to see the home she had painstakingly decorated during the last 30 years turn into a hospital. Helen also wanted Harry to have the best professional care provided around the clock. She found a long-term care site, and Harry was admitted to a licensed full-service residential care facility.

> Harry lives in the past. He thinks he should be going to work, and talks about going to play golf, which he has not played in several years. Although Harry still says words, his speech is unintelligible. He seems to be happy when around other people, but he cannot interact unless he receives one-to-one attention. Harry cannot dress himself even when given one article of clothing at a time. He needs someone to shave his face, and he can rinse his mouth but not brush his teeth. Harry still likes to walk, and he still has the physical capacity to ambulate without staff assistance. He has no perception of danger or others' privacy or personal space. He roams all over the facility and grounds unless carefully supervised. Harry interferes with the other residents by going into their rooms and rummaging through their belongings.

Harry Henley was in a new environment. When people with dementia are placed in a new environment, the goals in the care plan should be to facilitate adjustment, promote independence, and ensure safety. When he is roaming, Harry may be looking for his wife, trying to find his own room or the bathroom, or carrying out his usual, favored behavior pattern of walking. Because he has severe dementia, only familiar cues would be effective. Harry had lived with Helen in their home for 30 years and he was used to those surroundings, pictures, and furniture. New pictures and furniture lead to more confusion, and they do not provide the landmarks that he needs. Personal items are very important. Suggestions that would help Harry become oriented to his surroundings include the following:

- Furnish his room with his own furniture and personal belongings.
- Be sure that the door to his room contrasts with the color of the corridor walls and floor.
- Hang a picture of the Henleys, taken when they were first married, on his bedroom door.
- Be sure that the lighting does not cast shadows or cause glare that he could perceive as barriers to his room.

- Provide the same regularity in his daily routines that he was used to at home.
- Assign consistent staff so that Harry becomes accustomed to them.

Strategies to limit where Mr. Henley goes without physically restricting him include providing pleasant, inviting, and safe "on-limits" places for him to go; establishing walking paths with "dementia directions" for wayfinding; and providing outlets for his energy. The long-term care facility is the residents' "home." The environment should be homelike according to their perspectives. Although the term "day room" may be used among the staff, the more familiar term of "living room" or "family room" should be used when speaking with residents and visitors. Common areas should draw people with dementia into them by sensory appeal and the availability of leisure activities and hobbies (e.g., crafts, gardening, cooking, games). Mr. Henley should be accompanied to the living room activities so he will not stay only where he feels safe (e.g., in his room, around the nurses' station) or aimlessly wander through the facility.

Harry was accustomed to walking. To retain his capacity for independent ambulation and to prevent deconditioning, it is important for him to walk. Cues to help people with spatial disorientation find their way should be placed along the paths from residents' bedrooms to indoor and outdoor common areas. "Dementia directions" to help wayfinding in a residential facility include the following:

- Establishing for residents specific indoor and outdoor walking areas outlined with color-contrasting borders that clearly identify them as such
- Providing the correct amount of natural and artificial lighting to make the paths visible and appealing without casting shadows or causing glare
- Adding grab bars on the walls surrounding indoor paths
- Using pictures of familiar objects on the walls to identify the function of the common rooms (e.g., coffee cups on the way to the dining area, a picture of people sitting and socializing on the way to the living room)
- Removing anything that would interfere with a person's identifying the path for walking
- Providing areas for rest stops
- Assigning staff to provide guidance as needed

Although walking was previously his favorite pastime, Mr. Henley had been pursuing additional activities at home with his caregivers. Providing energy outlets is important for people with dementia across the disease continuum. Unfortunately, because of the fiscal considerations of long-term-care facilities, the one-to-one involvement that Harry received at home was not feasible.

Group approaches should be provided (see Chapter 6 for interventions to compensate for the inability to initiate meaningful activities).

Harry could be "lured" into the family room to participate in diversional activities that also stimulate the senses. Bright Eyes is a sensory experience exercise that is provided in a group setting to promote social interaction and to stimulate the senses (Trudeau, 1999; see also Chapter 6). The concept of "Bright Eyes" can be used in the following way. A CNA could greet Harry in the hall and say, "Harry, we're talking about what a great golfer Ben Hogan was. Come on in." The CNA gathers the residents and follows the occupational therapist's plan for "Golf Bright Eyes." The CNA follows the golf theme, arranges chairs so that residents sit in a circle, and helps invoke their senses as follows:

Olfactory—smell fresh grass clippings

Kinesthetic—take turns holding a putter and stroking a golf ball into a cup

Tactile—touch and pass around golf visors or astro-turf

Visual—look at posters of famous golfers or famous golf courses

Auditory—listen to a recording of crowd cheering or verbal reminiscence about famous golfers

Gustatory—drinking a nonalcoholic beer

## REFERENCES

Barr, R., & Foley, D. (1993). Driving with cognitive impairment. *Journal of the American Geriatrics Society, 41*, 889–891.

Greenwood, P.M., Parasuraman, R., & Alexander, G.E. (1997). Controlling the focus of spatial attention during visual search: Effects of advanced aging and Alzheimer's disease. *Neurosychology, 11*, 3–12.

Hirono, N., Mori, E., Ishii, K., Ikejiri, Y., Imamura, T., Shimomura, T., Hashimoto, M., Yamashita, H., & Sasaki, M. (1998). Hypofunction in the posterior cingulate gyrus correlates with disorientation for time and place in Alzheimer's disease. *Journal of Neurology, Neurosurgery and Psychiatry, 64*, 552–554.

Holden, J.E., & Therrien, B. (1989). The effects of hippocampal damage on adaptation to novelty in rats. *Journal of Neuroscience Nursing, 21*(1), 38–41.

Holden, J.E., & Therrien, B. (1993). Cue familiarity reduces spatial disorientation following hippocampal damage. *Nursing Research, 42*, 338–343.

Mendez, M.F., Cherrier, M.N., & Meadows, R.S. (1996). Depth perception in Alzheimer's disease. *Perceptual and Motor Skills, 83*(3, Part 1), 987–995.

Odenheimer, G., Beaudet, M., Jette, A.M., Albert, M., Albert, M.B., Grande, L., & Minaker, K.L. (1994). Performance based driving evaluation of the elderly driver: Safety, reliability and validity. *Journal of Gerontology, 49*, M153–M159.

Reinah, S.J. (1997). Driving with Alzheimer's disease: The anatomy of a crash. *Alzheimer Disease and Associated Disorders, 11*(Suppl. 1), 21–27.

Trudeau, S.A. (1999). Bright Eyes: A structured sensory stimulation intervention. In L. Volicer & L. Bloom-Charette (Eds.), *Enhancing quality of life for persons with advanced Alzheimer's disease* (pp. 93–106). Philadelphia: Brunner/Mazel.

# 9

# Resistiveness to Care

Mr. Ingram is a 74-year-old World War II veteran and a retired postal worker who was diagnosed as having Alzheimer's disease 3 years ago. His disease is now in a moderate to severe stage. He lives at home with his wife, who is his primary caregiver, and he receives care at the outpatient department of a nearby VA hospital. During an outpatient visit, Mrs. Ingram is asked by a nurse how things are going at home. She tells the nurse that her husband does not let her take him into the bathroom, so he is often incontinent of urine. The nurse asks Mrs. Ingram to describe her husband's behavior in more detail. She answers that he also refuses to be helped when his clothes need changing or he needs to shower, saying, "No, no, no!" When she persists, he adds loudly, "Don't you dare or I'll kill you!" Then he leaves the room, pulling away if she tries to hold him. The only way she can change him is to "tackle him to the floor." For him to take a shower, she has to go in with him, "clothes and all." Once his clothes are wet, he will take them off.

Mrs. Ingram confides that her husband's behavior frightens her and that she is exhausted and does not know how much longer she can care for him. Three adult children and seven grandchildren live down the street. Although they are "very involved and helpful," and have a "wonderful relationship" with Mr. Ingram, his wife says, "Everything changes when it's time to dress or bathe him. Why is he so angry when we are just trying to help?"

Resistiveness to care (RTC) encompasses the behaviors that are used by a person with dementia to withstand or oppose care. These behaviors are invoked and occur primarily during hands-on care. RTC can occur during any activity of daily living (ADL), including bathing, dressing, toileting, eating, walking, and administering medication. It also can occur when the caregiver attempts to redirect the person. RTC is a common behavioral consequence during the moderate to severe stages of dementia. RTC is a source of stress for both the individual and the caregiver. It is a major reason for institutionalization and the use of psychotropic medications and restraints. Consequences of RTC for the person with dementia include discomfort, increased medication use, stress, not receiving necessary care, and the potential for abuse. Consequences of RTC for caregivers include stress, increased time commitment and difficulty when providing care, personal injury, feelings of guilt or inadequacy, worry about making things worse, and depletion of psychological resources for caregiving.

## PROPERTIES OF RESISTIVE BEHAVIORS

A model for the behavioral dimensions of resistiveness and their parameters has been developed by the authors and associates (Mahoney et al., 1999) and is shown in Figure 9.1. Resistive behaviors are passive or active and include verbal and physical resistance to care. Specific behaviors used by the person with dementia are related to the disease stage. For example, people who are nonverbal may cry or use physical behaviors such as clenching their mouths or turning their heads away to resist taking a medication. People who have retained their mobility may try to move away from the caregiver. When an escape is thwarted, a person with dementia may respond with aggressive behaviors such as threatening or hitting. As with Mr. Ingram, several behaviors often are used to resist care. The number (*range*) and type (*active/passive*) of resistive behaviors represent both the person's capacity to mount a response and how threatening the situation is to the person. Often, a *pattern* of escalation can be identified. For example, Mr. Ingram said no several times before he threatened his wife and pushed her away. Although the "active" behaviors may command more attention, recognition of all resistive behaviors is important to understand RTC from the person's perspective and to plan treatment.

Frequency, duration, and intensity also are parameters of resistive behaviors. Assessment of these parameters provides important information about resistiveness. This information is useful in planning interventions and monitoring their effectiveness. *Frequency* refers to how often RTC occurs (e.g., daily

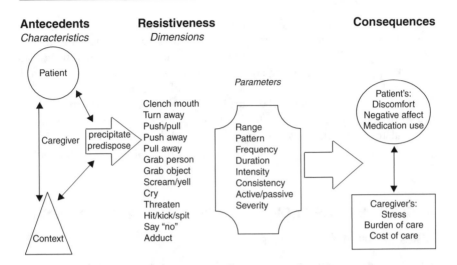

**Antecedents**
*Characteristics*

**Resistiveness**
*Dimensions*

**Consequences**

*Figure 9.1.    RTC model. (From Development and Testing of the Resistiveness to Care Scale, Mahoney, E.K., Hurley, A.C., Volicer, L., Bell, M., Gianotis, P., Hartshorn, M., Lane, P., Lesperance, R., MacDonald, S., Novakoff, L., Rheaume, Y., Timms, R., & Warden, V.,* Research in Nursing & Health, *Copyright ©1999 [Wiley-Liss, Inc., a subsidiary of] John Wiley & Sons. Reprinted by permission.)*

versus occasionally; during most care versus during only some ADLs). Mr. Ingram was resistive every day during two specific ADLs, bathing and dressing. *Duration* refers to the percentage of time during an ADL that resistiveness occurs and can be fleeting to constant. Mr. Ingram's resistive behaviors were of moderate duration, lasting from the initiation of care through the first several minutes. *Intensity,* the degree of force used, can range from mild to extreme. Behaviors of mild intensity may be barely noticeable, whereas those of extreme intensity are highly disruptive or disturbing. When the number of different resistive behaviors and their frequency, duration, and intensity are combined, the result is the *severity* of resistiveness. Therefore, decreasing the number, frequency, duration, or intensity of resistive behaviors reduces RTC severity.

A detailed assessment of resistiveness should include specific resistive behaviors and their parameters. The nurse in the case study began her assessment with open-ended inquiries such as "Think back on the most uncomfortable or difficult time you have had caring for your husband. Tell me about what happens when your husband needs to change his clothes." Follow-up questions should address specific behaviors and their frequency, duration, and intensity. Knowing what, when, and how is necessary to establish baseline assessment data and to develop short- and long-term goals. For example, short-term goals that indicate a clinically significant improvement for Mr. Ingram include 1) the frequency of resistive behaviors during bathing will decrease from daily to less than 3 times per week; 2) the resistive behaviors *turn away, pull away,* and *say no* are of short duration, lasting less than 1 minute; 3) the resistive behavior, *threaten,* is of mild intensity; and 4) Mr. Ingram will not experience RTC during dressing. By achieving any of these goals, the severity of RTC is reduced. The long-term patient goal (outcome) is minimal to no resistiveness during all ADLs while still receiving necessary care. The caregiver goal is to obtain a statement from Mrs. Ingram that she is able to manage RTC.

## ASSESSMENT OF PEOPLE "AT RISK" FOR RESISTIVENESS

### ABCs of Behavior Analysis

The nurse's assessment during the Ingrams' outpatient visit identified specific resistive behaviors. When resistive behavior occurred, the caregiver tried various strategies to manage it, noting their effectiveness and their impact on Mrs. Ingram's fear, fatigue, and frustration. These are examples of the "ABCs" of behavior analysis: antecedents, behaviors, and consequences. By using the ABC approach to assessment, it is possible to identify 1) what events and circumstances invoke resistiveness (antecedents), 2) the types and characteristics of resistiveness (behavior), and 3) outcomes that need immediate or long-term attention (consequences).

The characteristics of the person, the caregiver, and the context of care interact to predispose a person with dementia to resist care or to precipitate an actual episode of RTC (Figure 9.1). Behavioral scientists believe that all behavior has meaning (Eibl-Eibesfeldt, 1989). Resistiveness may be a symptom of an underlying process. It also may be a meaningful response to disability or a response to an environment that is perceived to be threatening, uncomfortable, confusing, or beyond control (Gwyther, 1994; Potts, Richie, & Kaas, 1996; Sloane et al., 1995). To learn what factors and circumstances actually invoke RTC, it is necessary to identify the antecedents.

In Mr. Ingram's case, RTC occurs after he has been incontinent and when Mrs. Ingram attempts to bathe and dress him. More detailed information about these antecedents are needed. For example, information about when and why Mr. Ingram is incontinent and how Mrs. Ingram attempts to help would be useful. When sufficient information is not available, however, it is still useful to know that Mr. Ingram is always resistive when he needs to be changed. Mrs. Ingram can be taught anticipatory problem-solving strategies.

The nurse suggests to Mrs. Ingram that she keep a diary (as a behavior log) and bring it with her to each clinic visit. Mrs. Ingram records resistive behaviors and their parameters and the contexts surrounding each instance of RTC. The diary provides documentation of the problems and progress in meeting goals and is used as a basis to revise the care plan. The nurse looks for patterns to identify key areas for intervention. For example, the diary reveals that Mr. Ingram becomes resistive when his wife unfastens his belt and unzips his pants. The nurse recommends giving Mr. Ingram sweat pants that he can manage by himself and using distraction techniques. For example, Mrs. Ingram can talk with her husband about his favorite dog while they walk to the bathroom. This lessens the focus on what he "has to do."

## VARIABLES IN PEOPLE WITH DEMENTIA

Personality and previous life experience may play a role in any behavioral symptom, including RTC (see Chapter 1). For example, one person might cry in response to feelings of frustration or lack of control, whereas another might lash out. Life patterns have an unpredictable influence on the dementing process. To provide insight into current behavior and what coping strategies to encourage, it may be helpful to know how the person with dementia coped with stress before onset of the disease.

Other variables that place people with dementia "at risk" for RTC can be seen in the model of behavioral symptoms of dementia presented in the Introduction. These variables include functional impairment, delusions, hallucinations, and depression. In Mr. Ingram's case there is insufficient assessment data to rule in or rule out these causes of RTC. For example, it is known that Mr. Ingram can walk independently and that he undresses himself in the shower when his clothes are wet. It is not known, however, whether he can no longer identify the bathroom (agnosia), communicate his needs with language (aphasia), or carry out a sequence of actions (apraxia). If he has a functional impairment that can be treated, then incontinence (antecedent) is decreased, his sense of control is maintained, and RTC is prevented. In another possible scenario, Mr. Ingram may experience delusions. In the case study his wife approached him to unzip and remove his pants. Mr. Ingram may have interpreted this action as a threat, which caused a "fight or flight" response and resulted in his threatening words and escape attempts. Another possibility is that Mr. Ingram is depressed and he reacted with anger (see Chapter 3). These actions are examples of resistiveness as a symptom of an underlying process. Interventions always should be guided by the assessment of underlying core processes because treatment of the primary consequences of dementia, which lead to peripheral symptoms, is more effective.

The variables discussed thus far—life pattern, functional impairment, delusions, hallucinations, and depression—are underlying processes that place people with dementia at risk for RTC. For people at risk, additional variables such as pain, fear, stress, or lack of control actually may invoke resistive behaviors (Algase et al., 1996). These behaviors need to be assessed by observing both verbal and nonverbal patient cues. For example, if people with dementia grimace, moan, and pull away every time their arms are moved, then they could be experiencing pain. If they hold on to the door frame, saying, "Don't go in there," every time they are led to the bathroom, then they could be experiencing fear. If resistiveness is worse when they are tired and agitated before an ADL begins, then they could be experiencing stress. If resistiveness occurs only during ADLs that require a great deal of assistance, then they could be defending against unwanted care. Although they have dementia, care recipients still may not agree with caregivers' timing or goals, and they may refuse help or care (Volicer, Hurley, & Mahoney, 1995). Thus, resistiveness may be an attempt to maintain some semblance of control.

## CAREGIVER VARIABLES

RTC does not occur in isolation, but rather in interaction among the person with dementia, his or her caregiver, and the environment (Figure 9.1). Some resistive behaviors are tied closely to the caregiver's behavior, which can range from soothing to distressing. For example, the difference between a person simply leaving a room versus actively pulling away from a caregiver may be related to whether the person is being held back. Relaxed and smiling caregiver behavior is related to calm and functional behavior on the part of older adults with dementia (Burgener, Jirovec, Murrell, & Barton, 1992).

When a person with dementia exhibits resistiveness, the caregiver's behavior needs to be evaluated. Some questions to ask include the following:

- Is the caregiver making demands that create stress or are beyond the ability of the person with dementia?
- Is the caregiver rushing through an ADL?
- Is the person being overstimulated by, for example, too many directions at a time?
- Do the caregiver's verbal and nonverbal communications convey respect for the person with dementia?
- Is the caregiver touching the person without warning in a manner that might be perceived as threatening or invasive?
- Is the caregiver doing something painful?
- Does the caregiver "take charge" rather than allow the person with dementia to maintain some control?
- Does the caregiver's own level of stress inhibit his or her ability to model calm and relaxed behavior?

Some of these caregiver variables may be well intentioned, motivated by a busy work schedule, or even inadvertent. Nonetheless, the way in which behaviors and interactions are perceived by the person with dementia is an important factor that affects his or her behavior.

Caregiver characteristics such as age and gender also can be important in ways that may or may not be anticipated. For example, a particular caregiver's characteristics may remind Mr. Ingram of a beloved grandchild or of a lifelong rival, and this attribute can affect both perception and behavior. Such information should be incorporated into the person's care plan.

## Context of Care

Recognition of the circumstances that are most likely to provoke resistive behaviors provides important clinical information. Some people are resistive during all ADLs, although it is more common for individual patterns to emerge. Mr. Ingram's resistiveness during bathing, dressing, and toileting illustrates his specific pattern. Measured across many ADLs and people with dementia, bathing elicits the greatest severity of resistiveness. It is important to be aware, however, that different ADLs are associated with different degrees of severity of resistiveness in different individuals. Assessing the ABCs of behavior analysis, with particular attention paid to patterns of RTC, helps the caregiver to anticipate and, ideally, prevent or minimize resistiveness.

Occasionally, behaviors such as screaming, grabbing, and hitting surprise the caregiver because they seem to come out of the blue. When these spontaneous behaviors are analyzed, it is found that most follow a stimulus such as a Hoyer lift moving upward, a whirlpool motor being turned on, the shock of skin first touching water, or being turned to the opposite side of the bed. Caregivers who mentally replay these unexpected resistive behaviors should gain insight into the world of the person with dementia, and they can help more effectively the next time around. In this regard, some practical and ethical questions to ask include the following:

- Is this care necessary?
- Is it necessary right now?
- What is the person feeling?
- Is my approach appropriate to those feelings?

ADLs range from least complex to most complex and follow a predictable pattern of regression during a progressive disorder such as Alzheimer's disease. The least complex ADL is eating and the most complex is bathing. It is not surprising, therefore, that bathing is the ADL that is associated most often with severe behavioral consequences. Not only does bathing involve performing and coordinating many steps but it is also more personal because it involves the person's entire, and naked, body. In addition, the water temperature may be too hot or too cold and there may be drafts in the bathing area. Many people with dementia are afraid of water, particularly when it strikes their head. Some clinicians have found that bedtime care is associated with a high incidence of resistiveness, perhaps because of its complexity and timing. Bedtime care combines dressing with toileting, washing, and perhaps mobility assistance. Other possible sources of resistiveness include "sundowning" (see Chapter 12) or the effect of fatigue or cumulative stress from the events of the day. For all of these reasons, a detailed assessment of the environmental context is an important part of assessing people "at risk" for resistiveness.

## SYMPTOM MANAGEMENT

Symptom management can be directed at the symptom (therapeutic) or at its etiology (preventive) (University of California, San Francisco School of Nursing Symptom Management Faculty Group, 1994). Even a hypothetical etiology is useful in planning individualized care. The goal is to decrease RTC frequency and duration and the numbers of resistive behaviors and their intensities. The following goals of care for the person with dementia have been identified: to feel safe, to feel physically comfortable, to experience a sense of control, to experience minimal stress, and to experience pleasure (Ryden & Feldt, 1992). Because fear, lack of pain control, anxiety, and stress are among the antecedents to resistiveness, these goals provide direction in planning care. Interventions such as promoting functional ability, controlling pain, and creating a comfortable, relaxed, caring, and safe-feeling environment prevent resistiveness by treating common etiologies.

RTC often is temporary, and the person with dementia may cooperate if the caregiver repeats the approach after a short period of time. This time period allows the person to forget that he or she did not want to cooperate (Volicer et al., 1995). Another effective strategy, which Mrs. Ingram used, is distraction. Taking the focus away from the caregiving activity by joking or talking may allow the person to cooperate.

### PREVENTION

The Ingrams' dilemma suggests the use of preventive strategies. For example, if Mr. Ingram's resistiveness is associated with incontinence, then prevention of incontinence could effectively eliminate resistive behavior associated with incontinence care. A toileting schedule could be established and accomplished while attention to other important antecedents is maintained.

Mrs. Ingram sees a pattern in her husband's behavior. He seems restless and fidgety before he is incontinent of urine, and this occurs at 4-hour intervals throughout the day. The nurse's suggestion that he wear sweatpants is working well because Mr. Ingram can manage them by himself. A toileting schedule of every 3½ hours is instituted. At the designated time, Mrs. Ingram guides Mr. Ingram into the bathroom in a calm, unhurried, and matter-of-fact manner while walking, talking, and smiling. She gives directions one step at a time and tries to keep her tone relaxed and pleasant. Sometimes, running water into the sink helps Mr. Ingram to urinate.

Mrs. Ingram reports that her husband uses the toilet approximately 75% of the time. When his clothes need to be changed, a calm and distracting approach reduces the range and intensity of resistive behaviors. Still, he often says, "no," but if Mrs. Ingram waits a few minutes and tries again, his behavior does not escalate. She now realizes that she had been overly insistent and tried to rush her husband through ADLs, thinking "quicker is better." The new approaches work in the familiar home environment, but Mr. Ingram is still resistive when he and his wife go out to visit people or go to the clinic. At these times, Mr. Ingram wears an incontinence brief that they refer to as "government underwear" to preserve his self-esteem.

Bathing practices need to be evaluated. Several useful approaches have been described by an interdisciplinary team of clinical experts in the care of people with dementia (Sloane et al., 1995). For example, simple bathroom modifications can make the environment more pleasant and less stressful (Table 9.1). A technique for bathing, "The Towel Bath," was designed by these experts to minimize known antecedents to resistive behaviors (Figure 9.2).

## BEHAVIORAL INTERVENTIONS

Several easy strategies are available to prevent or treat RTC. Sometimes, simply waiting a few minutes to perform care is the best approach. It is erroneous to think, "The sooner we get through this the better." Rushing through an

**Table 9.1.  Recommended environmental characteristics for bathing areas**

Make the room feel private and personal to the person with dementia.
Design the environment to keep residents warm.
Use music for residents who find it relaxing.
Adjust lighting so that it is soft (no glare).
Reduce the noise level.
Use homelike furnishings.
Use aromas to evoke memories, set mood, and make the bathing experience pleasant.
Make bathing equipment comfortable and functional.

Adapted from Sloane et al., 1995.

ADL to which the person is being resistive is invariably counterproductive. ADLs that can be scheduled, such as bathing, should be planned for times

---

*Equipment:*
2 bath blankets
Large plastic bag containing
– 1 large (6'6" × 3') lightweight towel, fan folded
– 1 standard bath towel
– 2 washclothes
2-quart plastic pitcher filled with bath temperature water (approximately 105° F), to which you

*Preparing the Resident*
Explain the bath. Make the room quiet or play soft music. Dim the lights if this calms the resident. Ensure privacy. Wash hands. If necessary, work one bath blanket under the resident to protect the bed linen and provide warmth. Undress the resident, keeping him or her covered with bed linen or the second bath blanket. You also may protect covering linen by folding it at the end of the bed.

*Preparing the Bath*
Pour the soapy water into the plastic bag, and work the solution into the towels and washcloths until they are uniformly damp but not soggy. If necessary, wring out excess solution through the open end of the bag into the sink. Twist the top of the bag closed to retain heat. Take the plastic bag containing the warm towels and washcloths to the person's bedside.

*Bathing the Resident*
Expose the resident's shoulders and upper chest, and immediately cover the area with the warm, moist large towel. Then gently and gradually uncover the resident while simultaneously unrolling the wet towel to re-cover the resident. Start washing at whatever part of the body is least distressing to the resident. For example, start at the feet and cleanse the body in an upward direction by massaging gently through the towel. Wash the backs of the legs by bending the person's knee and going underneath. As you move upward, roll the towel upward and cover the person with the bath blanket. After bathing the trunk, use the upper end of the towel to bathe the face, neck, and ears. You also may hand one of the washcloths to the resident and encourage independent face washing. Then turn the resident on his or her side and place the smaller warm towel from the plastic bag onto the back, washing in a similar manner, while warming the resident's front with the bath blanket. No rinsing or drying is required. Use a washcloth from the plastic bag to provide perineal care. Gloves should be worn when washing the perineal and rectal areas.

*After the Bath*
If it provides a relaxing break, allow the resident to remain unclothed and covered with the bath blanket and bed linen; dressing at a later time. A dry cotton bath blanket (warmed if possible) placed next to the skin and tucked close provides comfort and warmth. Place used linen into the plastic bag, tie the bag, and place it in a hamper.

---

*Figure 9.2.   The towel bath. (From Sloane, P.D., Rader, J., Barrick, A.L., Hoeffer, B., Dwyer, S., McKenzie, D., Lavelle, M., Buckwalter, K., Arrington, L., & Pruitt, T. [1995]. Bathing persons with dementia.* Gerontologist, 35, *675; reprinted by permission.)*

when the person is not fatigued. The behavior diary is useful for identifying patterns in daily rhythm when people are at their best, and this information should be included in the care plan. Redirection is used to channel a person's energy to another activity. For example, handing the person a washcloth and asking him or her to wash his or her face allows the caregiver to proceed with other parts of the bath and promotes the person's independence and personal control. Alternatively, simply giving the person something to hold, such as a colorful geometric-shaped ball with multiple handles, redirects the person from grabbing the caregiver. An occupational therapist should be consulted to fashion an object that is safe and useful for the person's level of function. Other behavioral interventions, which can be adapted to the person's functional ability and environment, are distraction, music, and Snoezelen (for more information on Snoezelen, see Chapters 6 and 7).

## Distraction

Distraction is useful to direct the person's attention away from the stressful stimulus. The particular approach depends on the severity of dementia and the number of available caregivers. Engaging the person in conversation on a favorite topic or reminiscing about happy memories that are retained takes the focus away from the task and places it on the person. This person-centered approach is effective even with people who have significant cognitive and language impairment (Hurley, 1999; Kovach & Meyer-Arnold, 1996). Distraction also facilitates the use of smiling, eye contact, and relaxed caregiver behaviors, which promote calm, functional behavior in people with dementia (Burgener et al., 1992). In an institutional setting, distraction is accomplished by using two caregivers. While one caregiver engages the person's attention by, for example, talking, reminiscing, joking, or singing, a second caregiver performs the ADL care. Distraction, when implemented according to these guidelines, is an effective strategy. A word of caution is necessary, however: The presence of two caregivers can create overstimulation and competing demands for the person with dementia if each person is giving directions, performing care, or even talking with the other caregiver. This is not the way to use distraction and must be avoided. Distraction is person centered and pleasant. As with all interventions, the response of the person to the intervention needs to be documented, and effective approaches should be included in the care plan for all to follow.

## Music

Research supports the use of classical and favored music to promote relaxation and improve behavior during ADLs in people with dementia. Both types of music improve mood. Whatever music is pleasurable to the person with dementia should be tried. The contemporary cohort of people with dementia grew up with big band music and popular songs from the World War II years through the 1950s. The family should be asked about the person's music preferences. Music played before ADLs promotes relaxation. Classical music played during mealtime and during bathing reduces behavioral symptoms, improves eating, and has the added positive benefit of improving quality of life for both the person with dementia and the caregiver (Goddaer & Abraham, 1994; Thomas, Heitman, & Alexander, 1997). When a person's favorite music is known, playing those pieces is more effective than playing general music (Gerdner, 1997). Singing favorite songs during bathing can be used as a part of reminiscing. Whether the effect of music is relaxation, distraction, or both, it works and needs to be used purposefully and consistently.

## PHARMACOLOGICAL INTERVENTIONS

Medications are an adjunct to, not a substitute for, nonpharmacological strategies to manage resistiveness. First, a careful assessment of baseline behavior is performed before the medication trial. Second, an ongoing assessment of behavioral responses to the medication is made. Finally, an assessment of side effects is carefully conducted and fully documented.

RTC can be precipitated by pain. Whenever possible, the cause of pain should be identified and eliminated. If the cause of pain cannot be prevented, as in, for example, arthritis, then it should be treated. Analgesics should be given prior to activities that cause pain. Arthritic pain is aggravated by stiffness from disuse, and this can be treated with gentle exercise supplemented with effective analgesia. Freedom from pain is essential for a good quality of life. The Discomfort Scale (Hurley, Volicer, Hanrahan, Houde, & Volicer, 1992) was developed specifically for the assessment of people with dementia and should be used to evaluate the effectiveness of the care plan in reducing pain.

> Mr. and Mrs. Ingram arrive at the hospital for an outpatient visit. Mr. Ingram's appearance is disheveled. His clothes are dirty and he smells of urine. His hair is uncombed. Mrs. Ingram has dark circles under her eyes and she is guarding her right arm, which has bruises in the shape of handprints. She states, "He didn't mean to hurt me. He would never hurt me." She then begins to cry. The nurse acknowledges Mrs. Ingram's feelings, provides immediate support, refers her to the caregiver support group at VA, and discusses respite care to break the cycle.
>
> On respite admission assessment, Mr. Ingram is found to have a badly sprained wrist from when he tried to break a fall 2 days earlier. A splint is applied and he is given an analgesic. During the week of respite, Mrs. Ingram has an opportunity to relax and to spend some time with her new granddaughter.

Some people with dementia, who consistently demonstrate RTC that does not respond to behavioral interventions and results in negative consequences for them, may benefit from a medication trial. If delusions or hallucinations (see Chapter 4) potentially contribute to resistiveness, then an antipsychotic medication trial may be appropriate. Another class of medications to be considered is antidepressants (discussed in Chapter 3). The person for whom such medications are prescribed must have a documented diagnosis for which that medication is warranted.

Sedation is a major side effect of many drugs that help decrease psychiatric symptoms. Antipsychotic medication can interfere with functional ability and participation in activities and may increase the risk of falling and functional dependence. If the adverse effects of a medication cause more difficulties than the problem for which it was prescribed, then the medication should be discontinued.

Another issue is that of scheduled medication doses versus "as needed" (PRN) doses. Because medicaton onset usually is longer than the activity to which the person is resistant, PRN medications have limited usefulness unless they are given in anticipation of resistiveness. The duration of drug action, indicated by its half-life, also is important because both therapeutic benefits and side effects will last beyond the length of the activity. The best approach for the person who requires pharmacological treatment is to time regularly prescribed medication doses so that the peak effect coincides with the timing of resistiveness. The class of drugs that usually is considered for PRN medication is the sedative-hypnotics, which are used to treat anxiety (see Chapter 7). Patterns of use must be examined to evaluate and revise the effectiveness of the standard medication regimen.

Mr. Ingram seems more comfortable, and he is sleeping well at night. He participates in the respite unit recreational activities and is even quite gregarious—except during morning care. His resistiveness escalates to combativeness when staff take him to the shower. He tries to leave the bathroom and often grabs and squeezes the nursing assistant's arm. His voice is heard all through the unit as he yells, "Stop it! Get away! I'm not like that! Get away from me!" These behaviors persist even when staff use distraction techniques and bathe him in bed. Mr. Ingram is diagnosed as having delusions, and risperidone, 0.5 mg/day, is prescribed. It is to be given at 8:00 A.M., followed by morning care at 9:00 A.M. Mr. Ingram's behavior stabilizes, and he has no side effects. He returns home after a week of respite care, still on this medication. The medication regimen will be reevaluated at his next clinic visit.

Regular examination of the medication regimen is important to evaluate continued therapeutic effect, continued need, and the presence of side effects that warrant discontinuation. Medications may serve a supporting role, but the goals of safety, comfort, a sense of control, minimal levels of stress, and optimal levels of pleasure are achieved with a total care environment that incorporates a full range of therapeutic strategies.

## REFERENCES

Algase, D.L., Beck, C., Kolanowski, A., Whall, A., Berent, S., Richards, K., & Beattie, E. (1996, November/December). Need-driven dementia-compromised behavior: An alternative view of disruptive behavior. *American Journal of Alzheimer's Disease,* pp. 10–19.

Burgener, S.C., Jirovec, M., Murrell, L., & Barton, D. (1992). Caregiver and environmental variables related to difficult behaviors in institutionalized demented elderly persons. *Journal of Gerontology: Psychological Sciences, 47,* P242–P249.

Eibl-Eibesfeldt, I. (1989). *Human ethology.* New York: Aldine de Gruyter.

Gerdner, L. (1997). An individualized music intervention for agitation. *Journal of the American Psychiatric Nurses Association, 3,* 177–184.

Goddaer, J., & Abraham, I.L. (1994). Effects of relaxing music on agitation during meals among nursing home residents with severe cognitive impairment. *Archives of Psychiatric Nursing, 8*(3), 150–158.

Gwyther, L. (1994). Managing challenging behaviors at home. *Alzheimer Disease and Associated Disorders, 8*(Suppl. 3), P110–P112.

Hurley, A.C. (1999). *Summary report: Protocols to manage resistiveness to care in veterans with Alzheimer's disease* (HSR&D grant NRI No. 96-023). Washington, DC: Department of Veterans Affairs.

Hurley, A.C., Volicer, B., Hanrahan, P.A., Houde, S., & Volicer, L. (1992). Assessment of discomfort in advanced Alzheimer patients. *Research in Nursing & Health, 15,* 369–377.

Kovach, C., & Meyer-Arnold, E.A. (1996). Coping with conflicting agendas: The bathing experience of cognitively impaired older adults. *Scholarly Inquiry for Nursing Practice, 10*(1), 37–42.

Mahoney, E.K., Hurley, A.C., Volicer, L., Bell, M., Gianotis, P., Hartshorn, M., Lane, P., Lesperance, R., MacDonald, S., Novakoff, L., Rheaume, Y., Timms, R., & Warden, V. (1999). Development and testing of the Resistiveness to Care Scale. *Research in Nursing & Health, 22,* 27–38.

Potts, H.W., Richie, M.F., & Kaas, M.J. (1996). Resistance to care. *Journal of Gerontological Nursing, 22*(11), 11–16.

Ryden, M., & Feldt, K.S. (1992). Goal-directed care: Caring for aggressive nursing home residents with dementia. *Journal of Gerontological Nursing, 18*(11), 35–41.

Sloane, P.D., Rader, J., Barrick, A.L., Hoeffer, B., Dwyer, S., McKenzie, D., Lavelle, M., Buckwalter, K., Arrington, L., & Pruitt, T. (1995). Bathing persons with dementia. *Gerontologist, 35,* 672–678.

Thomas, D.W., Heitman, R.J., & Alexander, T. (1997). The effects of music on bathing cooperation for residents with dementia. *Journal of Music Therapy, 34*(4), 246–259.

University of California, San Francisco, School of Nursing Symptom Management Faculty Group. (1994). A model for symptom management. *Image: The Journal of Nursing Scholarship, 26*(4), 272–276.

Volicer, L., Hurley, A.C., & Mahoney, E. (1995). Management of behavioral symptoms of dementia. *Nursing Home Medicine, 3*(12), 300–306.

# 10

# Food Refusal

A long-term care facility just received 24-hour notice that a surveyor from the state Department of Public Health will be making a site inspection for license renewal and will be reviewing records tomorrow. One of the unit's residents, Mrs. Jeng, and her care plan surely will be reviewed because she is underweight. This raises the question of whether Mrs. Jeng should have a permanent feeding tube placed to remedy the problem.

Mrs. Jeng is a 70-year-old widow who refuses food and has lost a great deal of weight since she developed dementia—15 pounds in the past 3 months. She weighs 90 pounds, which is only 70% of her ideal body weight according to the weight chart. Staff feel quite troubled that Mrs. Jeng will not open her mouth when they try to feed her. Now they fear that there will be problems because of the site visit. The issue of a feeding tube is being raised again. Last month the medical director wanted a feeding tube placed in Mrs. Jeng to decrease the risk of pressure ulcers and other complications related to malnutrition. Although her family and the nursing staff are concerned about Mrs. Jeng's continued weight loss, they are uncomfortable about trying to force feed her either by prying her mouth open or by using a feeding tube. Attempts at "encouraging increased intake" do not work, provoke resistiveness in Mrs. Jeng, and cause ambivalent feelings in staff, who are unwilling to coerce residents to do things against their wills. Yet all fear for Mrs. Jeng's well-being.

## GENERAL GUIDELINES TO PROMOTE EATING AND PREVENT FOOD REFUSAL

One important goal of care for individuals with dementia is to provide adequate nutrition by promoting eating and preventing food refusal. Although all individuals who have dementia are unique, and no single blueprint fits into all care plans, there are some general suggestions to help promote eating as the dementia progresses.

Three years ago, Mrs. Jeng was diagnosed as having mild dementia. She lived alone in a small congregate living facility apartment in the Asian community of a large West Coast city. She had tremendous social support from her own family of four married children and their families. Her family, however, shared knowledge of her memory loss and related problems with only a few close friends. Because of the belief that memory problems and confusion are part of the normal aging process and the specific Chinese cultural belief that, as one becomes old, it is natural for the person to change into a baby (Levkoff, Lui, Fung, Hinton, & Chang, 1998), available community support from the Chinese Golden Age Center was not requested. From a physical standpoint, Mrs. Jeng's health was quite good. She had chronic mild hypertension that was well controlled by a low-salt diet and a mild diuretic. Mrs. Jeng also had mild arthritis with back pain for which she took several daily doses of a generic nonsteroidal anti-inflammatory drug. Her family provided for her daily needs with occasional assistance from friends.

Her daughter Jin, who works in the city, was the primary caregiver. One day, when Jin was preparing for a family celebration, she bought her mother a new dress. When Mrs. Jeng tried the new dress on, Jin discovered that the dress size her mother usually wore was much too large. She realized that her mother had lost weight. Jin made an early-morning appointment for her mother for the following week at the neighborhood health center. She rescheduled her workday so she could accompany her mother to the evaluation.

Mrs. Jeng and Jin saw the nurse practitioner, who attempted to take a detailed history and performed a physical examination. Mrs. Jeng was unable to answer the health-related questions, and Jin could not answer many of the questions regarding food intake. Typically, Mrs. Jeng had meals and medications set up for her and then she ate alone. The nurse practitioner found no physical reason for Mrs. Jeng's weight loss and assessed that decreased food intake was the cause. The nurse discussed special eating issues in dementia with Jin and gave her some general rules for establishing a nourishment plan. The plan included planning food/nutrition/hydration, establishing eating areas, and facilitating the eating process.

## EATING PROBLEMS CAUSED BY DEMENTIA[1]

Specific eating issues that are related to food refusal occur during each of the progressive stages of dementia as a consequence of several primary or secondary symptoms or both. In all stages, however, changes in environment and disruption of usual routines can be upsetting to people with dementia, so mealtime rituals and consistency are helpful. One aspect of short-term memory loss for those with dementia is that they forget yesterday's menu or their most recent meal or snack. Although the caregiver may become bored with preparing the same food every day, the person with dementia will not become bored eating it. In fact, each meal and snack is a new experience. If the person likes a particular food, then it should be served. The same meals and snacks can be served until the person cannot eat them or does not want to eat them. At this point, the caregiver must reassess the person and his or her nutrition, and consider making modifications.

The nutritional plan should include consideration of the overall impact of dementia on the person. Dementia shortens the anticipated life span, and, thus, the medical management of other diseases should be based on a conservative approach. For example, although it is important for a young adult with diabetes to maintain good metabolic control to avoid late-stage complications, this is not a priority for people with dementia. Providing palatable food is more important than considering long-term risk factors that ultimately will not affect either survival or morbidity. Because many chronic diseases are common in older adults, it is likely that people with dementia will have other chronic conditions. Restrictive diets and multiple medications are not necessary unless they are required to alleviate troublesome symptoms. For instance, use of a low-salt diet to prevent the recurring symptoms of pulmonary edema may be required for one person who has congestive heart failure, but it may not be required for every older person with congestive failure or hypertension.

---

[1]The recommendations provided in this section were obtained from the clinical staff of the Edith Nourse Rogers Memorial Veterans Hospital Dementia Study Program in Bedford, Massachusetts (Warden, 1989); from the On-Line Learning Center (Smith, Gauthier, & Walker, 1998) of the Bedford Geriatric Research, Education and Clinical Center (GRECC), designed to help caregivers in the home; and from a videotape on teaching natural feeding strategies to caregivers of patients with late-stage dementia (Bedford GRECC, 1996).

A nutritional evaluation also should take into account that people with dementia may experience the same transient appetite-related symptoms as people without dementia. For example, anyone can have an "off day," but he or she may find that interest in food returns the following day.

## NOURISHMENT PLAN

The nutritional status of all older adults, especially older people with health problems, is so important that "weight is considered the 'fifth vital sign'" (Amella & Nurses Improving Care to the Hospitalized Elderly, 1998, p. 270). People with dementia are at risk for developing nutritional problems throughout the course of the disease (Frisoni, Franzoni, Bellelli, Morris, & Warden, 1998). Strategies to maintain adequate nutritional status should be put in place early in the disease process. Mealtimes should be made into focal points of the day, and other activities can be built around structured eating times. The primary caregiver should know the individual's current likes and dislikes, as well as his or her level of physical activity and degree of independence, and should identify how to make eating both pleasant and nutritious so that adequate calories, nutrition, and hydration are provided. A nourishment plan should specify which foods will be provided and how they will be prepared, identify the best environments in which to eat, and establish routines for the eating process.

### Planning Food/Nutrition

The primary caregiver should plan everything for the person with dementia well in advance (e.g., meal and snack times, food, utensils). Planning allows the caregiver to avoid interruptions once the meal begins so that all of the person's attention is focused on facilitating eating. To prevent distractions during the meal, caregivers can completely prepare the foods and beverages before setting them on the table (e.g., putting butter, salt, and sauces on food; putting sugar and cream in coffee). People with dementia can become distracted and unable to focus on more than one stimulus at a time. Therefore, caregivers can remove all other items from the table (e.g., flowers, napkin holder) to promote concentration on the task at hand. Food presentation, including colors and smell, is an important consideration. A low-fat/low-salt diet may not look or smell as appealing as a cheeseburger and French fries. Both smell and taste can stimulate a person's appetite. Because individuals in the later stages of dementia have a reduced life expectancy, considerations about "healthy heart" diets that are important earlier in life are of less concern. Also, some medications may be eliminated if their side effects alter the taste of food, diminish appetite, or interfere with the ability to use eating utensils.

Meal and snack times should be established to provide a stable routine. People with dementia are more focused and tend to be more cooperative in the morning after a good night's rest, so providing the bulk of the diet in the early part of the day works best. As the day goes on, they tire and become less able to stay focused. Instead of the traditional three meals of breakfast, lunch, and dinner, smaller and more frequent meals/snacks may promote eating.

The amount and type of food and beverages should be limited to prevent too much visual stimulation or too many choices, which can be overwhelming. Foods that are easily handled, chewed, and swallowed should be used. Small amounts of food, cut into small bites, work best, and softer, sweeter foods seem to be accepted more easily. Because people with dementia tend to lose weight later in the disease, it is important to maximize caloric density, unless they are above their ideal weight. Several foods have appealing characteristics and promote safe eating (Table 10.1).

Utensils may be misperceived by the person with dementia and can become safety hazards. In fact, the person may forget how to use them. Using finger foods is one way to address this problem. The use of one large spoon and a deep dish may suffice in the moderate through later stages of dementia.

## Establishing a Successful Environment for Eating

There is no one "right place" to eat. The area that works well is the best area for that individual, and the best area may vary with each meal. For example,

**Table 10.1.   Food characteristics to promote safe eating**

| Rationale / attributes | Examples of what to serve |
| --- | --- |
| Easy to eat | |
| Minimal chewing needed | Cooked vegetables, ground meat, boneless fish and chicken, crushed fruits, pancakes, soft rolls, macaroni and cheese, French toast |
| Finger foods | Toast, French fries, scrambled eggs in a pita pocket |
| Appealing | |
| Soft and smooth | Pureed fruits, puddings, casseroles, mashed potatoes with gravy, instant breakfast with whole milk or cream |
| Sweet tasting | Ice cream, popsicles, addition of vanilla syrup or fruits to yogurt |
| | **What to avoid** |
| Foods that may cause choking | |
| Chewy foods | Chewing gum, hot dogs, taffy |
| Crumbly foods | Doughnuts, crackers, nuts |
| Thin, watery liquids | Water, tea, soda |

sitting at the table for the breakfast meal, then holding a sandwich while walking about at lunch, may work for one person. Conversely, eating while moving may be contraindicated for a person who paces and may put an entire sandwich into his or her mouth at once, thus risking aspiration. A third person might eat well only when sitting down in a quiet spot. The behavior diary mentioned in Chapter 9 may help guide caregivers in determining an individual's "best area."

A comfortable, attractive dining area is important for people with early dementia. Caregivers should strive for a homelike or restaurantlike atmosphere for people with mild or moderate dementia. In the later stages of dementia, a simple table without linens, placemats, knives, decorations, butter, condiments, or paper napkins is appropriate. Some general tips are to design the dining area to avoid clutter on the table; remove anything from the table that can distract from eating, be confused with food, or cause an injury; and not serve steaming hot beverages or very hot food.

## Shaping the Eating Process

Several "do's and don'ts" promote eating and decrease the risk of food refusal and make eating satisfactory for both the person with dementia and the caregiver:

- Always have someone sitting at the table with the person during mealtimes. A caregiver eating at the same time can model the eating process.
- Avoid overstimulation. Turn off the television. Ask family and friends not to visit during mealtimes.
- Promote a pleasant eating situation. Try playing soothing music (Denney, 1997).
- Avoid interruptions once the meal has begun. Bring the person to the bathroom before the meal. At home, turn off the ringer on the telephone during the meal. Present only one food at a time to keep the person focused and to prevent playing with food.
- Do not give medications during meals because this can be distracting and alter the taste of food.
- Encourage independence, but try not to overwhelm the person. For example, say something or demonstrate what the person should do to begin eating (this may be necessary because of apraxia and agnosia; see Chapter 2). It helps to give simple, one-step commands, for example, "Take your spoon. Put the potatoes on the spoon. Put the spoon in your mouth. Chew the food. Swallow the food."
- Provide positive feedback. Praise the person for eating his or her meal.

Jin had to leave for work after she brought her mother back to her apartment, but she left lunch on the table. She also decided she would return for the dinner meal. Jin believes that she is a good caregiver, but she felt guilty when she was unable to answer the nurse practitioner's questions about Mrs. Jeng's day and her recent history. Jin wanted to find out why Mrs. Jeng was not eating as well as she had been, and she wanted to follow the nurse practitioner's advice about sitting with and assisting her mother during meals. When Jin began to eat dinner with Mrs. Jeng, she was surprised to see just how little her mother ate.

## MANAGING FOOD REFUSAL THROUGH PROGRESSIVE STAGES

Specific factors predispose individuals to food refusal through the progressive stages of dementia. Although cognitive and functional losses and psychiatric symptoms are the primary reasons, the caregiver/staff member or the eating environment may contribute to food refusal. During the course of dementia, individuals require increasing assistance with eating. Caregivers, however, should provide only as much assistance as necessary to prevent excess disability and to preserve people's remaining independence. People with dementia tend to lose abilities in the reverse order in which they were learned. Eating is one of the first behaviors learned by an infant; thus, some degree of eating ability is preserved through the end stages of the dementing illness.

The four stages of dementia presented in the Introduction help to characterize its progressive nature and establish foci for care, but no two human beings are alike. Dementia does not manifest itself uniformly across all individuals, even in identical twins with dementia. In some cases an individual may demonstrate some food-refusal behaviors that are typical of one stage only, whereas another person may demonstrate behaviors that cross several stages and require a variety of management strategies.

### Mild Dementia

Food refusal usually is not a problem in mild dementia. If the person with dementia is also depressed, however (see Chapter 3), then loss of appetite may result, and the primary symptom of depression should be treated. The person with mild dementia who refuses to eat may not have appetizing meals. Once the primary caregiver has prepared an easy-to-eat meal, the person with mild dementia should be able to eat independently. Help with meal setup, such as opening milk cartons, preparing coffee, and seasoning food, is needed.

### Moderate Dementia

Chapters 2 and 6 discuss some of the "A" complications (dementia symptoms that begin with the letter "A") that predispose people to food refusal in this stage. A person with moderate dementia may not recognize a fork as an eating tool (agnosia); may lose the ability to recognize food (agnosia) and attempt to eat nonfood items; may forget to eat (amnesia); may be unable to say what he or she likes or wants (aphasia); and may be unable to initiate the steps of scooping food onto an eating tool and bringing it to his or her mouth (apraxia).

Even though the physical ability to hold an eating tool, sit erect, and move one's arm is still intact in moderate dementia, the person with dementia will need help to start and complete the activities of eating. Caregivers need to provide the appropriate amount of assistance with eating and drinking. In the moderate and severe stages people need help during the meal and should not eat alone. To foster optimal independence, family members and staff should assist by being present and making the eating experience pleasurable by smiling and encouraging eating; helping the person to get started by having all food and beverages ready to eat and drink (e.g., by removing covers, by pouring liquids into a cup); offering finger foods; presenting one food at a time; and using only one utensil, such as a tablespoon.

## Severe Dementia

Resistiveness to care (see Chapter 9) and eating difficulties are the major causes of food refusal in people with severe dementia. The anticholinergic effects of neuroleptic medications for treating agitation or resistiveness can relax the muscles involved in swallowing (Frisoni et al., 1998). In this stage people with dementia may simply forget how to eat, chew their food for an excessively long time, or hold food in their cheeks (pouching). Caregiver help during eating is needed to provide careful supervision, cueing (reminding the person to eat, to chew, and to swallow), direct assistance, or complete feeding. Typically, some eating ability is preserved until very late in the disease. Eight years after the onset of dementia, approximately 50% of people still have significant eating ability (Volicer et al., 1987).

## Terminal Dementia

In the terminal stage, when individuals are confined to bed, mute, dysphagic, and subject to intercurrent infections, eating difficulties can become problematic (Volicer et al., 1989). The terminal stage of dementia is marked by great difficulty in swallowing (dysphagia) as a result of brain pathology that causes a loss of muscle coordination that is associated with progression of the dementia. People in the terminal stage of dementia must be fed. Choking, which may appear in the severe to terminal stages, can be prevented or at least minimized by avoiding thin liquids; feeding the person in a sitting position or keeping the head of the bed at a 90° angle; and using foods in which the texture of the bolus has sufficient moisture content to help passage through the pharynx and facilitate swallowing (Frisoni et al., 1998).

## PREVENTING/BREAKING THE CYCLE
## OF BEHAVIORS USED TO REFUSE FOOD

Loss of appetite may cause people to refuse to eat or to eat very little during all stages of dementia. It is common for individuals to have a few "off days" when they eat less, but they soon regain their appetite. Causes of appetite loss and food refusal can be evaluated to help manage specific causes (Table 10.2).

Some common factors directly cause food refusal or indirectly worsen the problem (e.g., depression, self-care deficit; see Chapters 3 and 5). Underlying health problems may remain undiagnosed because people in the later stages of dementia cannot report symptoms of a physical problem that is related to loss of appetite and food refusal. Sometimes the first symptom of an infection can be a change in behavior with loss of appetite. People with dementia can develop anorexia similar to that seen in individuals with terminal cancer or ketosis secondary to fat metabolism associated with weight loss.

As individuals become more dependent on caregivers, they require skilled attention to their unique feeding difficulties to ensure adequate nutrition. Caregivers must have time for and the system must support the individual needs of people who initially refuse food. It takes time to sit and make eye contact, chat, and make eating a pleasurable experience for people with dementia, and it is one of the most important components of long-term institutional care (Kayser-Jones & Schell, 1997). Skill and patience are required to use the right amount of coaxing and avoid the type of pressuring that leads to resistiveness (see Chapter 9).

As a result of the meeting with the nurse practitioner, Jin "loosened up" on Mrs. Jeng's low-salt diet and began preparing traditional Chinese foods that her mother particularly liked. Mrs. Jeng gained a little weight, but a few weeks later she fell in her home and was rushed to an acute care facility. The X-ray revealed a broken hip, which was successfully repaired. Mrs. Jeng's hospital stay, however, was not as successful as her surgery. The new environment, strange faces and noises, and the discomfort in her hip all contributed to increasing her confusion. She also was physically restrained to her bed. Two weeks after her hip fracture, Mrs. Jeng was transferred to a long-term care facility for rehabilitation. She arrived there in a confused and deconditioned state. She refused to eat and would not feed herself or open her mouth when staff tried to feed her.

People use many behaviors to refuse food. In one study of eating difficulties in a long-term care setting, 36 of 71 residents (51%) refused food (Volicer et al., 1989). During attempts at feeding, 89% of these residents turned their heads away when food was offered, 78% kept their mouths shut, 72% pushed

## Table 10.2. Managing food refusal

| Causes or predisposing factors | Interventions |
| --- | --- |
| Resident | Caregiver must assess cause or causes, develop care plan, and implement care plan |
| **Physical reasons** | |
| Fatigue | Look for signs of problems that are secondary to or unrelated to the dementia |
| | Daytime naps, drowsiness, wakefulness during the night—Establish care plan to promote night-time sleep |
| Overstimulation | Many visitors, increase in activities—Control stimulation, omit caffeine, promote longer sleep time |
| Not feeling well | Lethargy—Anyone can have an "off day"; provide lighter foods (milkshakes) |
| Constipated/impaction | Hard abdomen, no recent bowel movement—Common problem, use low-stimulation laxative; prevent with osmotic laxative (e.g., lactulose) |
| Other illness | Fever or change in behavior—Same incidence of other illness in older adults; identify and treat |
| Nausea | Possible drug side effect—Discontinue medication; change timing of medication administration |
| Dehydration | Decreased fluid intake—Choking on thin liquids and providing caloric dense nutrition may predispose; assess by symptom observation (e.g., dry mouth, furrowed tongue, possible tenting of forehead) |
| **Oral disease problems** | |
| Mouth | Look for indications of problems |
| | Examine mouth and teeth—Provide good mouth care; keep mouth clean; fix problem/painful teeth; treat gum disease |
| Ill-fitting dentures | Repair or fit for new dentures; use pureed diet |
| **Anorexia** | Treat underlying causes |
| Depression | Consider low-dose antidepressant |
| Ketosis | Give sweet foods |
| Side effects of medications | Discontinue or substitute drugs that do not alter taste or interfere with eating ability |
| Loss of appetite stimulus | Use sensory appeal (e.g., olfactory)—Try the smell of freshly baked bread with lunch |
| **Lost ability from dementia** | Promote independence without exceeding the person's ability; assist only as needed |
| Amnesia | Forgetting to eat meals; put food nourishment out; tell person, "It's lunchtime" |
| Apraxia | Initiate the eating process; hold your hand over person's hand on the spoon to start the process |
| Agnosia | Model the step, hand eating tool to person, "Here's your spoon," "Here's your cereal" |

| | |
|---|---|
| ADL deficit | Ready the meal for easy eating; use a deep plate and one large spoon; assist as needed |
| Coordination | Facilitate function of muscles that control chewing and swallowing; stroke cheek and throat |
| Short attention span | Keep focused on eating; remind person to "open, chew, swallow" |
| Unable to swallow | Remind person to "open, chew, swallow" independently |

**Staff members** — **Remember that eating is a critical ADL and important quality-of-life issue**

| | |
|---|---|
| Inadequate time | Plan adequate time; all staff help feed at meals; staff should eat before or after resident meal times |
| Inadequate knowledge | Interdisciplinary team planning, staff education, general feeding strategies for patients |
| Preferences | Learn person's food preferences and provide them; variety is not important |
| Feeding strategies | Establish eye contact, smile; coax using caloric-dense foods; add sweet to tip of spoon |
| Feeding myths | Tube feeding is not a panacea for food refusal (e.g., can cause aspiration pneumonia) |
| Oral feeding advantages | Preserves taste of food and provides pleasure at mealtimes |

**Environment** — **Make social, physical, and caregiving environments conducive to dining and pleasurable eating**

| | |
|---|---|
| Chaotic or noisy dining area | Divide large area into small sections; play soothing music |
| Food | Individualize to person's ability and preferences |
| Unappealing | Provide food the person likes and can eat; do not restrict diet |
| Wrong composition | Cut into small mouthfuls, and avoid thin liquids or crumbs that may cause choking |
| Tray | Make a special presentation unique for each person |
| Too much food | Try a sandwich or half a sandwich at a time |
| Improper utensils | Use only one eating tool (spoon in later stages) |

the utensil or hand away, and 39% spit out food. Yet, after refusing to be fed during mealtime, 44% ate independently afterward when finger food was left for them. Some interventions for preventing the food refusal cycle and what to do if these behaviors appear have been developed (Table 10.3).

It is important to formulate an individual care plan for each resident of a long-term care facility. An interdisciplinary team approach to solving the potentially multiple problems that underlie food refusal brings together perspectives from several disciplines to resolve the problem. Representatives from each discipline—nurse, dietitian, occupational therapist, physician, pharmacist, and possibly a dentist—should conduct a discipline-specific assessment based on their unique contributions to the total care plan. Individualized culture-based information should be obtained from families and each resident's medical record. For Mrs. Jeng, for example, the team should know answers to questions such as the following: Was she born in America? What

**Table 10.3.    Preventing/breaking cycle of behaviors used to refuse food**

| Challenging behaviors | Suggested approaches for staff |
|---|---|
| **Passive** | **Provide sensory stimulation to engage patient** |
| Unaware of environment | Auditory: "Hello"; "Here's your lunch"; "It smells good" |
| | Olfactory: Provide aroma of food product (e.g., freshly baked brownies) |
| | Visual: Smile and make eye contact |
| | Tactile: Move hand over person's hand to take spoon |
| | Taste: Put small amount of sweet food on lips |
| No involvement with feeder | Hold hand and make eye contact |
| "Kisses the spoon" | Place food on person's lips for him or her to lick off |
| **Defensive** | **Gently encourage to carry out eating behaviors** |
| Will not go to dining area | Hold individual's hand and guide to eating area, saying, "Come with me—we'll eat now" |
| Walks away from dining area | Wait, then guide individual back to area; set up eating area next to the individual |
| Averts head | Say person's name; engage; say, "Here's some pudding" |
| Closes mouth | Smile and say, "Open" |
| Clamps down on eating tool | Stroke cheek and say, "Eat" |
| Says, "I don't want to eat" | Divert; wait |
| Will not swallow | Stroke throat and say, "Swallow" |
| **Active opposition** | **Do not force; distract; wait** |
| Pushes utensil away | Distract from utensil; try again |
| Pushes feeder away | Stop; wait; come back later; leave finger food |
| Spits out food | Stop; wait |
| Screams "No!" | Stop; wait; distract; come back later |

language did she speak at home? What are her special dietary needs and preferences? Because food refusal is not a new problem, answers to additional questions should be obtained: How has this problem been managed before? What previous causes were identified? Which interventions were tried? Which interventions have been successful?

The team should then meet, share assessments made from each discipline's perspective, and collaborate to establish the initial care plan guidelines (Tables 10.2 and 10.3). They also should discuss Mrs. Jeng's target body weight. She weighed 104 pounds when she was admitted to the hospital after breaking her hip. She is 5 feet 3 inches tall, has a small body frame, and now weighs 90 pounds. People who are basically sedentary lose muscle mass (Khodeir, Conte, Frisoni, & Volicer, 1997). Mrs. Jeng spends her day sitting in a chair and, therefore, does not use many calories.

The plan should specify how to manage the behaviors that Mrs. Jeng uses to refuse food, establish objective and measurable goals, and set target dates for goal attainment. Because Jin is the primary family caregiver, she must have some input into establishing care goals. If possible, Jin should attend the interdisciplinary team meeting. Otherwise, an alternate method to include her input, such as through discussion with Mrs. Jeng's care manager, must be established. Family input to the care plan creates a therapeutic alliance, promotes communication, and provides practical advice for professionals. Family members can share residents' food likes and dislikes with staff. In this way, residents can be provided the meals that they prefer. For example, while Mrs. Jeng was at home, Jin changed her mother's diet so that it was more liberal with salt and was able to provide foods that Mrs. Jeng likes. Conversely, a resident's tastes can change, and a previous gourmet may come to like simple foods sweetened with yogurt. Staff should communicate such changes in food preference to the family.

If the eating/feeding problem or problems persist, then the person should be reassessed and the care plan adjusted. Medications may need to be added. For example, if Mrs. Jeng is depressed and the cause of her food refusal is loss of appetite, then low-dose sertraline should improve both her depression and appetite (Volicer, Rheaume, & Cyr, 1994). For anorexia associated with dementia, dronabinol may be considered as an appetite stimulant (Volicer, Stelly, Morris, McLaughlin, & Volicer, 1997).

Jin attended the team meeting and shared her mother's food preferences with the staff. The dietitian was able to modify Mrs. Jeng's diet and included more rice and foods resembling traditional Chinese food. Once Mrs. Jeng was presented with these dishes, her appetite improved and she began to eat her meals. Several months later, however, Mrs. Jeng refused to eat even her previously favorite foods and she lost more weight.

## PREVENTING THE CONSEQUENCES OF FOOD REFUSAL IN THE TERMINAL STAGE OF DEMENTIA

Many clinical issues in dementia care are complex and include ethical and legal components. The issues surrounding care for people with advanced dementia in the severe or terminal stage are highly complex. Especially difficult are the issues regarding initiation or withdrawal of a feeding tube. The initial question posed in this chapter was, "Should Mrs. Jeng have a permanent feeding tube?" Using a feeding tube, staff could be sure that Mrs. Jeng received exactly what was prescribed; she could gain weight if she was able to tolerate sufficient volume of the nutrients. The state surveyor could not fault the facility if a gastrostomy tube were placed. However, there are many disadvantages to a permanent feeding tube, such as the loss of the taste of food, the minimal interaction with a caregiver at mealtime, the need for physical restraints to prevent removal of the tube, and the complications that are associated with using the feeding tube (Volicer, Rheaume, Riley, Karner, & Glennon, 1990).

There are also widely held misconceptions about feeding tubes (Ahronheim, 1996, pp. 380, 382, 384, 385): "Tube feeding is ordinary care, like spoon feeding ... tube feeding is indicated in patients with aspiration pneumonia ... swallowing evaluations can identify patients who should receive tube feeding ... withholding or withdrawing ANH [artificial nutrition and hydration] leads to a painful death." Evidence from scientific clinical research has shown each of these misunderstandings to be incorrect (Ahronheim, 1996). Except for its symbolism, tube feeding does not resemble eating or drinking in any way, and it is associated with many potential complications. No evidence exists that any form of tube feeding reduces the risk of pneumonia, and there are a number of reasons why tube feeding may actually increase its risk. Even the diagnosis of "swallowing difficulties" is imprecise and of limited clinical value because interpretations of bedside swallowing evaluations and videofluoroscopy are subjective, and the techniques that are used to make these evaluations differ significantly from the normal physiologic function of swallowing. Dying without tube feeding is a natural process. There is much indirect evidence that terminal dehydration is not uncomfortable, and there is direct evidence from the observation that hospice patients regularly and volitionally reject food and water in the terminal phases of their illness.

The interdisciplinary team should meet again to review Mrs. Jeng's health status to determine her target body weight. The team should make a careful assessment for all of the potential causes of Mrs. Jeng's current food refusal and revise her care plan accordingly. In most cases eating difficulties can be managed by dietary, nursing, and medical strategies (Volicer, 1998).

Jin attends another family conference at which advantages and disadvantages of tube feeding are discussed. She decides she does not want to expose her mother to the discomfort and complications of tube feeding. She decides to enroll Mrs. Jeng in a hospice program. The hospice treatment plan recognizes the terminal nature of Mrs. Jeng's illness and acknowledges that weight loss during this stage of dementia is inevitable. The surveyor reviews Mrs. Jeng's care plan and does not find any problem with its implementation.

## REFERENCES

Ahronheim, J.C. (1996). Nutrition and hydration in the terminal patient *Clinics in Geriatric Medicine, 12,* 379–391.

Amella, E.J., & Nurses Improving Care to the Hospitalized Elderly (NICHE). (1998). Assessment and management of eating and feeding difficulties for older people: A NICHE protocol. *Geriatric Nursing, 19,* 269–275.

Bedford Geriatric Research, Education and Clinical Center. (1996). Alzheimer's disease: Natural feeding techniques (Color videotape) [Abstract]. *Gerontologist, 36* (Special Issue 1), 292.

Denney, A. (1997, July). Quiet music: An intervention for mealtime agitation? *Journal of Gerontological Nursing,* 16–23.

Frisoni, G.B., Franzoni, S., Bellelli, G., Morris, J., & Warden, V. (1998). Overcoming eating difficulties in the severely demented. In L. Volicer & A. Hurley (Eds.), *Hospice care for patients with advanced progressive dementia* (pp. 48–67). New York: Springer.

Hurley, A.C., Volicer, L., Warden, V., Smith, S.J., Glennon, M., Morris, J., & Whitaker, J. (1995). [Video]. *Alzheimer's disease: Natural feeding techniques.* (Distributed by Terra Nova Films, 9848 S. Winchester Avenue, Chicago, IL 60642.)

Kayser-Jones, J., & Schell, E. (1997, July). The mealtime experience of a cognitively impaired elder: Ineffective and effective strategies. *Journal of Gerontological Nursing,* 33–39.

Khodeir, M., Conte, E., Frisoni, G.B., & Volicer, L. (1997). Effect of decreased mobility on body composition in patients with Alzheimer's disease [Abstract]. *Gerontologist, 37,* (Special Issue 1), 85.

Levkoff, S., Lui, B., Fung, S., Hinton, L., & Chang, K. (1998). The evolution of a culturally distinct support group for Chinese caregivers of dementia-impaired elders: Trial and error. *Discussions on Caring, 1*(2), 47–82.

Smith, S., Gauthier, M.A., & Walker, R. (1998). *Eating and meals* [Online]. Available: http://www.xfaux.com/Alzheimer/Feeding/html

Volicer, L. (1998). Tube feeding in Alzheimer's disease is avoidable. In B. Vellas, S. Riviere, & J. Fitten (Eds.), *Research and practice in Alzheimer's disease: Weight loss & eating behaviour in Alzheimer's patients* (pp. 71–74). New York: Springer.

Volicer, L., Rheaume, Y., & Cyr, D. (1994). Treatment of depression in advanced Alzheimer's disease using sertraline. *Journal of Geriatric Psychiatry and Neurology, 7,* 227–229.

Volicer, L., Rheaume, Y., Riley, M.E., Karner, J., & Glennon, M. (1990). Discontinuation of tube feeding in patients with dementia of the Alzheimer type. *American Journal of Alzheimer's Care and Related Disorders and Research, 5,* 22–25.

Volicer, L., Seltzer, B., Rheaume, Y., Fabiszewski, K.J., Herz, L.R., Shapiro, R., & Innis, P. (1987). Progression of Alzheimer-type dementia in institutionalized patients: A cross-sectional study. *Journal of Applied Gerontology, 6,* 83–94.

Volicer, L., Seltzer, B., Rheaume, Y., Karner, J., Glennon, M., Riley, M.E., & Crino, P.B. (1989). Eating difficulties in patients with probable dementia of the Alzheimer type. *Journal of Geriatric Psychiatry and Neurology, 2,* 169–176.

Volicer, L., Stelly, M., Morris, J., McLaughlin, J., & Volicer, B. (1997). Effects of dronabinol on anorexia and disturbed behavior in patients with Alzheimer's disease. *International Journal of Geriatric Psychiatry, 12,* 913–919.

Warden, V.J. (1989). Waste not, want not. *Geriatric Nursing, 10,* 210–211.

# 11

# Insomnia

Sleep is necessary for the survival of all animals and humans and requires active involvement of the brain. Brain activity is different in the alert state compared with the sleep state, and it can be monitored by an electroencephalogram (EEG), which records electrical waves resulting from nerve cell stimulation.

## SLEEP STAGES

From EEG recordings, we can distinguish four different types of waves of differing frequency: beta, 14–25 cps (cycles per second); alpha, 8–13 cps; theta, 4–7 cps; and delta, 0.5–3 cps. Alpha and beta waves have low amplitudes (voltages), whereas delta and theta waves have larger amplitudes. Alpha waves occur during relaxation with eyes closed. The onset of sleep is marked by the disappearance of alpha waves. Other EEG characteristics that occur during sleep include *sleep spindles* (bursts of EEG waveforms of 11.5–16 cps) and *K complexes* (short bursts of high amplitude often followed by a spindle). According to EEG characteristics and eye movements, it is possible to distinguish five sleep stages (Table 11.1). Sleep Stages 1 and 2 can be considered a light sleep, whereas Stages 3 and 4 are deep, or slow-wave, sleep. Dreaming occurs mainly during the fifth stage of sleep, called rapid eye movement (REM) sleep.

**Table 11.1. Sleep stages**

| Stage | Predominant EEG waves | Eye movments |
|-------|----------------------|--------------|
| 1 | Mixed frequency, low voltage | Slow rolling |
| 2 | Sleep spindles and K complexes | Absent |
| 3 | Sleep spindles and slow waves | Absent |
| 4 | Mostly slow waves | Absent |
| REM | Mixed frequency, low voltage | Rapid |

REM, rapid eye movement.

After falling asleep, an individual progresses through Stages 1–4. Slow-wave sleep may alternate between Stages 3 and 4 and eventually is replaced by a REM sleep episode. Slow-wave sleep and REM sleep alternate approximately every 90–120 minutes. Sleep stages vary during normal sleep and may be punctuated by periods of awakenings. In young adults nightly percentages of each sleep stage are 2%–5% in Stage 1, 45%–55% in Stage 2, 3%–8% in Stage 3, 10%–15% in Stage 4, and 20%–25% in REM sleep. Less than 5% of the sleep time is spent "awake" (Hirshkowitz, Moore, Hamilton, Rando, & Karacan, 1992). Most deep sleep occurs during the first part of the night, and most REM sleep occurs during the second half of the night. The quality of sleep can be determined by examining sleep characteristics: 1) total sleep time; 2) latency to sleep; 3) number of awakenings; 4) sleep efficiency (total sleep time divided by time in bed); 5) latency to REM sleep; and 6) REM sleep length.

## REGULATION OF SLEEP

The ability to fall asleep varies during the 24-hour day. The major episode of sleepiness occurs typically in the evening. The approximately 24-hour cycle persists even when individuals are kept at a constant level of light with no environmental cues. This indicates the existence of an endogenous clock that regulates sleep and waking and also influences other bodily functions. This clock is called circadian (from the Latin *circa*, or about, and *dies*, or day) and is regulated by a group of cells in the hypothalamus called the suprachiasmatic nucleus (SCN). Other functions influenced by the SCN include regulation of body temperature, blood pressure, heart rate, hormonal secretion, motor performance, and cognitive performance. Sleep is tied closely to changes of body temperature. Healthy individuals become sleepy in the evening when their body temperatures decline and awaken in the morning after their body temperatures start to rise. The SCN also regulates secretion of some hormones, such as glucocorticoids, thyroid-stimulating hormone, and melatonin. There are other hormones that are not regulated by the SCN (e.g., growth hormone, prolactin) that are tied to the onset of sleep.

Prolonged wakefulness produces increased sleepiness. People who go to sleep after being awake for a long time will sleep longer, compensating for a sleep "debt." This sleep debt is specific for the type of sleep; for example, when individuals are deprived of REM sleep, they usually will have more REM sleep during the following nights. Studies that encourage subjects to sleep when they are inclined to do so indicate that human sleep may not be monophasic because subjects often sleep for a short period of time (1–2 hours) in the afternoon, in addition to a long night sleep (Campbell & Zulley, 1985). Thus, an afternoon nap may be promoted by an endogenous mechanism.

In young, healthy individuals the endogenous circadian rhythm usually is longer than 24 hours but it is adjusted to a 24-hour cycle by environmental cues, mainly light. Many blind people have circadian cycles that are longer than 24 hours and experience sleep difficulties when trying to maintain 24-hour routines. Morning light causes a shortening of the cycle (*phase advance*), which helps to maintain 24-hour rhythmicity. Other mechanisms that produce phase advance include secretion of pituitary adenylcyclase-activating peptide, which acts during the day; melatonin, which acts during the evening; and acetylcholine, which acts during the night (Gillette, 1997). All of these mechanisms are necessary for the maintenance of normal sleep. In contrast, exposure to evening light causes prolongation of the cycle (*phase delay*). The circadian rhythm also is influenced by the administration of psychoactive drugs such as benzodiazepines, which cause phase advance, and lithium, which causes phase delay.

The endogenous circadian rhythm depends on the activity of several genes that produce specific proteins. These proteins are transferred into the nuclei of SCN cells, where they inhibit the genes that are necessary for their own production. This inhibition generates a negative feedback loop that results in a cyclical activity of the SCN cells. Abnormality of one or more genes involved in this negative loop leads to the shortening of the circadian period of motor activity in hamsters and abnormal circadian rhythms in fruit flies (Gillette, 1997). Genetic regulation of circadian rhythms detected in animals indicates that genetic factors also may influence circadian rhythms and sleep behavior in humans.

Mr. Kupfer is a 72-year-old retired machinist who developed difficulties sleeping. He started waking early in the morning and could not go back to sleep. His wife, Kathy, also observed that he was napping during the day and was less interested in his hobbies. Mr. Kupfer visited his primary physician, who suggested lifestyle changes to improve his sleep. The physician recommended decreasing napping; maintaining a regular sleep–wake schedule; avoiding caffeine, nicotine, and alcohol in the evening; and avoiding exercise and exciting or emotionally upsetting activities close to bedtime.

## EFFECTS OF AGE ON SLEEP

Slow-wave sleep begins to decline after adolescence and eventually may disappear with advancing age (Hirshkowitz et al., 1992). Total sleep time also declines with aging, and sleep becomes increasingly intermixed with periods of wakefulness. This sleep change is called sleep fragmentation. Older adults often wake up earlier in the morning and take more daytime naps than younger individuals. Animal experiments indicate that these changes may be due to age-related dysfunction of the SCN (Gore, 1998). A decreased size and number of nerve cells containing vasopressin in the SCN are found in elderly individuals (Swaab, Fliers, & Partiman, 1985). Aging also decreases the amplitude of circadian melatonin secretion, resulting in lower total melatonin release and an earlier peak of melatonin secretions (phase advance) than in younger individuals. The differences of core body temperature during the day (amplitude of the circadian rhythm) are lower in elderly than in younger individuals, but the timing of the peak and nadir are not affected by age (Gore, 1998). This activity results in the uncoupling of melatonin secretion from body temperature rhythm, which may be mediated by a loss of the hypothermic effect of melatonin in elderly individuals. The sleep of older adults also may be disturbed because of an increased incidence of sleep-related motor disorders (SRMDs) and sleep-related respiratory disorders (SRRDs) (Figure 11.1).

> Mr. Kupfer's sleep improved somewhat after he made the lifestyle changes that were suggested by his physician. His wife, Kathy, however, began to complain about his snoring. The snoring awakened her and she was unsuccessful in stopping the snoring by making him roll over. Kathy also observed that Mr. Kupfer sometimes holds his breath while sleeping. Mr. Kupfer also believed that there was something wrong. He often felt tired in the morning and had a headache after awakening. He reported his snoring and other symptoms to his physician. The physician ordered a sleep laboratory examination, which found that Mr. Kupfer has sleep apnea, with significantly reduced oxygen concentration in his blood during the apneic episodes. The sleep laboratory physician recommended that Mr. Kupfer start using nasal continuous positive airway pressure (CPAP) treatment.

### SLEEP-RELATED RESPIRATORY DISORDERS

Disordered breathing during sleep is quite common in elderly individuals. The SRRDs consist of periodic breath holding during sleep (sleep apnea) that is accompanied by snoring and daytime sleepiness. Sleep apnea decreases blood oxygen content and increases the risk of hypertension and the risk of death

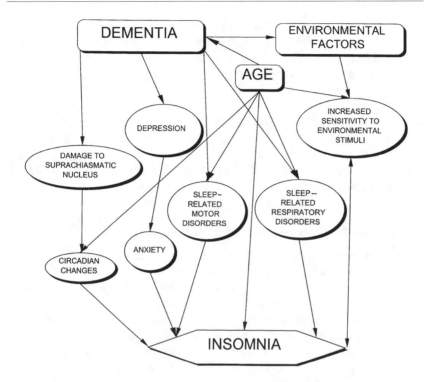

*Figure 11.1.   Factors contributing to insomnia in elderly individuals.*

during sleep (Bliwise, 1997). SRRDs also may be a risk factor for stroke. In individuals older than age 65, at least mild SRRDs occur in 24% of independently living older adults, 33% of acutely hospitalized older adults, and 42% of nursing facility residents (Ancoli-Israel et al., 1991b).

The prevalence of SRRDs increases with age. Self-reported snoring has been estimated to occur in about 30% of men and 20% of women at age 40, and the prevalence increases to 50% of men and 40% of women at age 60. This increased prevalence of snoring may be related to the age-related increase in pharyngeal resistance and mouth ventilation. Pharyngeal resistance also is increased by alcohol, and this effect is more pronounced in older individuals. Another risk factor for SRRDs is obesity, which may be more significant in women than in men (Bliwise, 1993).

## SLEEP-RELATED MOTOR DISORDERS

The most common of the SRMDs is periodic leg movements. The incidence of SRMDs increases with age, and they are estimated to occur in 45% of independently living elderly individuals (Ancoli-Israel et al., 1991a). SRMDs may be related to age-related decline of dopamine receptors, because L-dopa and dopamine receptor agonists decrease the number of periodic leg movements. Other possible precipitating factors include osteoarthritic changes, venous insufficiency in the lower extremities, and iron-deficiency anemia (Bliwise, 1993).

SRMDs are more common in people with Parkinson's disease, osteoarthritis of the hips or lower limbs, restless leg syndrome, and fibromyalgia. An epidemiological study of community-living older adults found that approximately one third of periodic leg movement episodes (on the average, 5.5/hour of sleep) resulted in arousal and that this arousal occurred in 22.6% of individuals (Bliwise, 1997).

## MEDICAL CONDITIONS COMMON IN OLDER ADULTS

A variety of medical conditions and medications that are used for the treatment of common medical conditions experienced by older people may lead to sleep disruption. Individuals using a health care system for any reason are more likely to report insomnia than individuals who are not using a system. Specific medical conditions that disrupt sleep include renal diseases, gastrointestinal illnesses, respiratory diseases, chronic pain, fibromyalgia, and menopause. Elderly individuals are more likely to be awakened by factors external to sleep (e.g., noise) than are younger individuals in the same stage of sleep. This tendency is aggravated by the decrease of slow-wave deep sleep with aging. Therefore, even low intensity of pain caused by symptoms of a disease, as well as other stimuli (e.g., full bladder), will result in disturbed sleep.

> Mr. Kupfer tried to use CPAP, and his wife noticed that he was not snoring. He also felt more rested in the morning and no longer had headaches, but he was bothered by the mask and the noise of the machine. He continued to use the CPAP, but only intermittently and not for the whole night. Kathy was able to sleep better, but noticed that Mr. Kupfer was becoming quite forgetful. He had to write down all of his appointments and often forgot what he wanted to buy when he went shopping. He also did not remember information that Kathy told him, and he asked the same questions repeatedly. On one of his shopping trips, Mr. Kupfer got lost driving home, although he has lived in the neighborhood for 25 years. Kathy went with her husband to see his physician and reported the problems. The physician ordered laboratory tests and a detailed neuropsychological examination. He made a diagnosis of probable Alzheimer's disease. He prescribed donepezil (Aricept) for Mr. Kupfer to take in the evening.

# EFFECT OF DEMENTIA ON SLEEP

A retrospective evaluation of patients with autopsy-confirmed Alzheimer's disease found that disturbances of circadian rhythms were present in 56%, and the average time of onset of these disturbances was several months before the diagnosis of Alzheimer's disease (Jost & Grossberg, 1996). Disruptions of circadian rhythms observed in Alzheimer's disease include changes of sleep, body temperature, melatonin secretion, and possibly other physiological functions.

## STAGES OF SLEEP

EEG evaluation of sleep parameters in healthy controls and people with Alzheimer's disease in different stages of dementia show that several of these parameters change with the progression of dementia (Prinz et al., 1982). These progressive changes include decreased dominant frequency of EEG waves, decreased slow-wave and REM sleep, increased number and duration of nighttime awakenings, and increased REM latency. Other investigators also described decreased K complex and sleep spindle density (Montplaisir, Petit, Lorrain, Gauthier, & Nielsen, 1995).

These EEG findings are supported by monitoring circadian motor activity in controls and people with Alzheimer's disease. Individuals with Alzheimer's disease have a higher percentage of nocturnal activity than controls, corresponding to the clinical picture of fragmented sleep (Satlin, Volicer, Stopa, & Harper, 1995). The variation in motor activity during the day (circadian amplitude) is smaller in people with Alzheimer's disease than in controls, and the time of the maximal activity (*acrophase*) is delayed compared with controls. This phase delay also is observed in the circadian rhythm of core body temperature. In addition, melatonin secretion is decreased in people with Alzheimer's disease (Morita, Uchida, & Okamoto, 1996). These changes are probably caused by degenerative changes in the SCN that are more pronounced than changes that are caused by normal aging (Swaab et al., 1985).

## SLEEP-RELATED DISORDERS

Another cause of increased sleep disturbance in people with Alzheimer's disease is a higher incidence of SRRDs and SRMDs than in controls (Bader, Turesson, & Wallin, 1996). Sleep disturbances also occur in other forms of dementia, including multi-infarct dementia (Aharon-Peretz et al., 1991) and Parkinson's disease (Bliwise, 1997), and they may be even more severe than in Alzheimer's disease.

Mr. Kupfer's forgetfulness improved with the administration of Aricept, but he started having nightmares that woke him up. His physician recommended that he take donepezil in the morning instead of at night, and Mr. Kupfer's sleep improved. After a few months, however, Mr. Kupfer stopped watching television and was not interested in visiting his friends. His appetite decreased and he lost 15 pounds in 2 months. Mr. Kupfer complained of being tired all of the time and of feeling hopeless. He was waking early in the morning and was unable to go back to sleep. His primary physician referred him for a psychiatric evaluation. The psychiatrist made the diagnosis of depression and prescribed sertraline (Zoloft).

Donepezil is a drug that inhibits the breakdown of acetylcholine and delays the progression of cognitive changes in Alzheimer's disease (see Chapter 1). Nightmares in patients treated with donepezil can be prevented by changing the time of donepezil administration.

## EFFECTS OF DEPRESSION AND ANXIETY ON SLEEP

Depression and anxiety are other possible causes of sleep disturbances in people with Alzheimer's disease. Development of depression in people with dementia occurs often (see Chapter 3), and anxiety is a common symptom (see Chapter 7). Most EEG changes are similar in depressed and anxious individuals. These changes include increased sleep-onset latency, increased wake time after sleep onset, decreased total sleep time, decreased sleep efficiency, and decreased slow-wave sleep. The differences between depression and anxiety involve Stages 1 and 2 and REM sleep. Individuals suffering from anxiety have increased Stages 1 and 2 sleep and unchanged REM sleep, whereas depressed individuals have unchanged Stages 1 and 2 sleep, decreased REM latency, and increased REM sleep (Ware & Morin, 1997). Decreased REM sleep latency is proposed to be a biological marker for depression, but it also may occur in some people with generalized anxiety disorder.

The most common sleep-related symptom in depression is early-morning awakening, and a decrease in depressive symptomatology is associated with a decrease in early-morning awakening (Rodin, McAvay, & Timko, 1988). It also is possible, however, that insomnia increases the risk of depression and anxiety disorder. In an epidemiological study investigating the prevalence of psychiatric disorders individuals reporting persistent insomnia are more likely to report depression and anxiety at a follow-up interview 1 year later than are individuals whose insomnia has resolved (Ford & Kamerow, 1999). This finding suggests that the development of depression and anxiety may be prevented by the timely and effective treatment of insomnia.

Sleep deprivation increases irritability and pain sensitivity, and it results in memory impairment, including diminished immediate recall and decreased long-term memory (Ware & Morin, 1997). Individuals who are not depressed develop mild depressive symptoms following sleep deprivation, whereas sleep deprivation produces an antidepressant effect in some depressed individuals. This effect is short lasting, and depressive symptoms return even after a short nap. The antidepressant effect is mediated by the suppression of REM sleep.

> Two weeks after the initiation of antidepressant therapy, Mr. Kupfer's appetite improved and he again became interested in his hobbies and friends. He was able to sleep longer in the morning, but his memory did not improve. He continued to forget what he was told and began experiencing problems finding the right words when speaking. Mr. Kupfer also gradually lost the ability to use tools and read newspapers. About a year later, he developed difficulty falling asleep and was sometimes up for the whole night. Kathy was not able to sleep when he was awake and became exhausted. She took Mr. Kupfer to see his physician, who prescribed trazodone (Desyrel) to be taken before going to sleep; the administration of sertraline was continued in the morning.

## TREATMENT OF INSOMNIA

Several strategies are useful when people with dementia experience insomnia: lifestyle changes, behavioral strategies (stimulus control, sleep-restriction therapy), chronobiological strategies (light therapy, increasing daytime physical activity, passive heating), and pharmacological treatment. As Mr. Kupfer's case demonstrates, several of these strategies may have to be used in the same individual.

### LIFESTYLE CHANGES

Lifestyle change is the first intervention to explore with all individuals to establish proper sleep hygiene. Daily activities that are inconsistent with the maintenance of high-quality sleep and daytime alertness are taking daytime naps; spending too much time in bed; keeping irregular sleep–wake schedules; being inactive; routinely using products that interfere with sleep (e.g., caffeine, nicotine, alcohol); scheduling exercise close to bedtime; engaging in exciting or emotionally upsetting activities close to bedtime; and having a poor sleep environment (e.g., uncomfortable bed; bedroom too bright, hot, cold, noisy, or stuffy) (Bootzin & Rider, 1997).

Some studies report that sleep hygiene recommendations improve sleep, and 70% of those who try the recommendations report that they are helpful

(Hauri, 1999). A meta-analysis of studies that evaluated nonpharmacological treatments for insomnia found that sleep hygiene recommendations, as a sole intervention, are not as effective as other treatments (Morin, Culbert, & Schwartz, 1994). Therefore, sleep hygiene recommendations should be combined with behavioral techniques and other interventions if necessary.

## BEHAVIORAL STRATEGIES

Some behavioral strategies are effective in cognitively intact individuals but are not useful in individuals with dementia. For example, cognitive therapy requires people with dementia to learn specific strategies such as paradoxical intention, cognitive restructuring, thought stopping, and articulatory suppression (Bootzin & Rider, 1997). Similarly, relaxation training, meditation, and biofeedback require a degree of personal involvement and commitment that cannot be achieved by an individual with cognitive impairment. However, two methods—stimulus control and sleep-restriction therapy—can be applied in the early stages of dementia by a dedicated caregiver.

### Stimulus Control

Stimulus control is designed to help the person establish a consistent sleep–wake rhythm, strengthen the bed and bedroom as cues for sleep, and weaken them as cues for activities that may interfere with sleep. Bootzin, Epstein, and Wood (1991, p. 25) developed the following instructions for stimulus control:

1. Lie down intending to go to sleep only when you are sleepy.
2. Do not use your bed for anything except sleep; that is, do not read, watch television, eat, or worry in bed. Sexual activity is the only exception to this rule. On such occasions, the instructions are to be followed afterward, when you intend to go to sleep.
3. If you find yourself unable to fall asleep, get up and go into another room. Stay up as long as you wish and then return to the bedroom to sleep. Although we do not want you to watch the clock, we want you to get out of bed if you do not fall asleep immediately. Remember, the goal is to associate your bed with falling asleep quickly! If you are in bed more than about 10 minutes without falling asleep and have not gotten up, you are not following this instruction.
4. If you still cannot fall asleep, repeat Step 3. Do this as often as necessary throughout the night.
5. Set your alarm and get up at the same time every morning irrespective of how much sleep you get during the night. This will help your body to acquire a consistent sleep rhythm.
6. Do not nap during the day.

Several studies indicate that these stimulus control instructions constitute one of the most effective single-component therapies for insomnia (Morin et al., 1994). Application of this strategy in individuals with dementia, however, is not easy (Table 11.2). It requires significant involvement of a caregiver to monitor the person's sleep, be able to get him or her up during the night if the person is not sleeping, get him or her up at the same time every day, and prevent napping during the day.

### Sleep-Restriction Therapy

Sleep-restriction therapy is based on the observation that many people with insomnia spend too much time in bed attempting to sleep. The aim of this therapy is to consolidate sleep by restricting the amount of time spent in bed to the person's estimated average length of nighttime sleep (Spielman, Saskin, & Thorpy, 1987). This restriction induces partial sleep deprivation with daytime sleepiness at the beginning of the treatment. No matter how little a patient sleeps at the beginning of the treatment, the prescribed sleep window is always a minimum of 4.5 hours. Sleep-restriction therapy is effective in cognitively intact individuals (Morin et al., 1994), but intense involvement of the caregiver is necessary to apply this strategy to individuals with dementia. This therapy should be used with caution when applying it to people with dementia because discouraging older people from daytime napping is reported to exacerbate their fatigue. It also increases agitated behaviors of individuals with dementia without improving their nighttime sleep (Cohen-Mansfield & Werner, 1995).

## CHRONOBIOLOGICAL STRATEGIES

The regular sleep–wake cycle is a result of normal circadian rhythms of several body functions. Circadian rhythms are regulated by nerve cells contained in the SCN and are affected by environment influences such as light level, activ-

**Table 11.2.   Application of stimulus control strategies to individuals with dementia**

Do not get the individual into bed too early in the evening.

Prevent the individual from lying in bed during the day by keeping the bedroom door closed if necessary.

If the individual does not fall asleep in 10–15 minutes, then allow him or her to get up; provide meaningful activities.

If the individual is waking up because of the need to urinate, then restrict evening intake of liquids and make sure he or she voids before going to bed.

Wake the individual at the same time every morning regardless of when he or she went to sleep.

Keep the individual occupied with a meaningful activity during the day to prevent napping.

ity, and food intake. The circadian rhythm generated by the SCN is longer than 24 hours. However, environmental influences, especially light, shorten this rhythm in healthy individuals and synchronize it with the 24-hour day.

Alzheimer's disease causes nerve cell death in many areas of the brain, including the SCN. The cell loss in the SCN leads to abnormalities of circadian rhythms in people with Alzheimer's disease. These abnormalities include prolongation of the circadian rhythm and desynchronization between different physiological functions, such as body temperature and motor activity (Satlin et al., 1995). People with Alzheimer's disease also have increased motor activity during the night, which indicates a less effective sleep pattern with frequent periods of wakefulness. If insomnia in a patient with Alzheimer's disease is related to circadian rhythm disturbance, then improvement of circadian rhythms may result in improved sleep. Several strategies may affect circadian rhythms: light therapy, increase in daytime physical activity, and passive heating to increase body temperature.

## Light Therapy

Light exposure is the most important environmental influence affecting circadian rhythms. The effect of light exposure depends on the light intensity, duration, and proximity of exposure to the time of lowest body temperature (nadir). A bright light exposure administered before the nadir prolongs the circadian cycle, whereas an exposure after the nadir shortens the circadian cycle. The closer to the nadir that the exposure occurs, the greater its effect on the circadian rhythm. In healthy individuals the nadir occurs early in the morning before awakening, but in some individuals with Alzheimer's disease the nadir occurs after the person is awake (Satlin et al., 1995). Thus, in healthy individuals, morning light shortens circadian rhythm and synchronizes it with the 24-hour day, whereas in some people with Alzheimer's disease, morning light leads to prolongation of the circadian rhythm.

Light therapy is effective in the treatment of seasonal affective disorder and insomnia in cognitively intact elderly people (Cooke, Kreydatus, Atherton, & Thoman, 1998). This finding led to several studies investigating the effect of light therapy in Alzheimer's disease and other progressive dementias. In most of these studies morning or evening exposure to bright light resulted in improved sleep and decreased daytime agitation (Harper, Rheaume, Manning, & Volicer, 1999). The duration of light exposure usually is 2 hours, and in some studies morning light exposure was more effective than evening light.

The administration of light therapy in individuals with dementia poses some problems. Some individuals may be unwilling to sit in front of a light box or wear a visor that is equipped with a light source. Use of restraints would affect the person's behavior and may be unethical. A room with a uniformly high level of lighting, in which the person can move freely and engage in activities, allows light treatment of unrestrained agitated individuals (Rheaume, Manning, Harper, & Volicer, 1998). An increased level of lighting in chronic care facilities may be beneficial for sleep and behavior disturbances. In one study increased light exposure during the day improved some parameters of motor activity circadian rhythm in people with Alzheimer's disease, but it did not affect blind individuals (Van Someren, Kessler, Mirmiran, & Swaab, 1997).

## Increasing Daytime Physical Activity

Changes in activity level affect circadian rhythms in laboratory animals. Forced bed rest disturbs body temperature rhythm in humans (Van Someren, Mirmiran, & Swaab, 1993). Fitness training improves subjective sleep quality of elderly individuals, but it is not clear whether this effect is mediated by a change of circadian rhythms. A physical activity program during the daytime did not improve sleeping patterns of individuals with dementia (Alessi et al., 1995).

Acute exercise improves sleep if it is performed a few hours before going to bed. Strenuous exercise, which increases body temperature, is required to achieve this effect. The effect of exercise is probably mediated by an increase in body temperature because cooling of the body during exercise blocks the effect of exercise on sleep (Van Someren et al., 1993).

## Passive Heating

Few individuals with dementia are able to engage in strenuous exercise that would increase their body temperature. In young adults, however, a body temperature increase induced by passive heating increases slow-wave sleep to essentially the same extent as exercise (Van Someren et al., 1997). A bath at 41°C for 15–30 minutes increases body temperature by 2°C, increases plasma melatonin levels, and improves sleep. The best time for this bath is late afternoon or early evening, because heating earlier in the day is ineffective and heating just before going to bed may disrupt sleep. All of the studies exploring the effect of passive heating, however, were done with healthy young adults, and it is not clear how applicable these findings are to elderly individuals with dementia. It also may be difficult to apply this technique to people with dementia who are often resistive during bathing (see Chapter 9) and do not understand the need for an extended bath time.

## PHARMACOLOGICAL TREATMENT

Even with the advances in nonpharmacological strategies for the treatment of insomnia that were described earlier, many individuals with insomnia require pharmacological treatment. Hypnotics, such as benzodiazepines or zolpidem (Ambien), are drugs of choice in the treatment of insomnia in cognitively intact individuals. These medications, however, should be avoided in individuals with dementia if possible. Benzodiazepines often cause daytime sedation and increase the risk for falls and aspiration. They also may cause worsening of memory deficit and can lead to increased agitation shortly after administration (paradoxical reaction) or even the next day. There is some evidence that sundown syndrome may be related to a delayed effect of hypnotics, because individuals exhibiting sundown syndrome are more likely to be receiving chloralhydrate (Little, Satlin, Sunderland, & Volicer, 1995). Benzodiazepines and other hypnotics are not intended to be administered for an extended period of time, but insomnia in individuals with dementia usually is chronic and requires long-term therapy. For all of these reasons, alternate pharmacological agents for the management of insomnia in individuals with dementia should be considered.

Either of the two primary consequences of dementia, depression and delusions/hallucinations, may cause insomnia in individuals with dementia. Insomnia is a symptom of depression in cognitively intact individuals and responds well to antidepressant therapy. In individuals with dementia it is sometimes necessary to use sedating antidepressants to prevent nighttime behavioral symptoms. Sedating antidepressants include doxepin (Adapin, Sinequan) and trazodone. Doxepin blocks acetylcholine receptors and therefore may produce significant adverse effects that include dry mouth, urinary retention, and increased risk of delirium. Trazodone is much safer, although it may lead to dystonia, postural hypotension, and, rarely, priapism. Trazodone is not a potent antidepressant, however, and it must be combined with other antidepressants for effective therapy.

> Mr. Kupfer's sleep improved after trazodone was initiated. One year later, however, he again started to get up early in the morning, get dressed, and leave the house. Kathy was not able to get enough sleep and became exhausted from trying to keep him in the house. Mr. Kupfer was examined by a visiting nurse, who found that he believes he is still working and must be at his job in the mornings. Mr. Kupfer was seen by his psychiatrist, who prescribed risperidone (Risperdal). Mr. Kupfer stopped trying to leave the house, and his sleep improved.

Delusions are another possible cause of sleep disturbances. Neuroleptics, usually in low doses that do not cause sedation, are effective in blocking delusions and hallucinations (see Chapter 4). Although some neuroleptics are sedating (e.g., thioridazine), they should not be used in high doses to promote sleep. In people with dementia who are depressed and experience delusions or hallucinations, combined treatment with an antidepressant and a neuroleptic often is necessary. Risperidone and olanzapine (Zyprexa) are drugs of choice for people with dementia and depression because they affect mood less than do the typical antipsychotics.

## REFERENCES

Aharon-Peretz, J., Masiah, A., Pillar, T., Epstein, R., Tzischinsky, O., & Lavie, P. (1991). Sleep-wake cycles in multi-infarct dementia and dementia of the Alzheimer's type. *Neurology, 41*, 1616–1619.

Alessi, C.A., Schnelle, J.F., McRae, P.G., Ouslander, J.G., Al Samarrai, N., Simmons, S.F., & Traub, S. (1995). Does physical activity improve sleep in impaired nursing home residents? *Journal of the American Geriatrics Society, 43*, 1098–1102.

Ancoli-Israel, S., Kripke, D.F., Klauber, M.R., Mason, W.J., Fell, R., & Kaplan, O. (1991a). Periodic limb movements in sleep in community dwelling elderly. *Sleep, 14*, 496–500.

Ancoli-Israel, S., Kripke, D.F., Klauber, M.R., Mason, W.J., Fell, R., & Kaplan, O. (1991b). Sleep disordered breathing in community dwelling elderly. *Sleep, 14*, 486–495.

Bader, G.G., Turesson, K., & Wallin, A. (1996). Sleep-related breathing and movement disorders in healthy elderly and demented subjects. *Dementia, 7*, 279–287.

Bliwise, D.L. (1993). Sleep in normal aging and dementia. *Sleep, 16*, 40–81.

Bliwise, D.L. (1997). Sleep and aging. In M.R. Pressman & W.C. Orr (Eds.), *Understanding sleep: The evaluation and treatment of sleep disorders* (pp. 441–464). Washington, DC: American Psychological Association.

Bootzin, R.R., Epstein, D., & Wood, J.M. (1991). Stimulus control instructions. In P.J. Hauri (Ed.), *Case studies in insomnia* (pp. 19–28). New York: Plenum.

Bootzin, R.R., & Rider, S.P. (1997). Behavioral techniques and biofeedback for insomnia. In M.R. Pressman & W.C. Orr (Eds.), *Understanding sleep: The evaluation and treatment of sleep disorders* (pp. 315–338). Washington, DC: American Psychological Association.

Campbell, S.S., & Zulley, J. (1985). Ultradian components of human sleep/wake patterns during disentrainment. In H. Schulz & P. Lavie (Eds.), *Ultradian rhythms in physiology and behavior* (pp. 247–272). Berlin: Springer-Verlag.

Cohen-Mansfield, J., & Werner, P. (1995). Environmental influences on agitation: An integrative summary of an observational study. *American Journal of Alzheimer's Care, 10*(1), 32–39.

Cooke, K.M., Kreydatus, M.A., Atherton, A., & Thoman, E.B. (1998). The effect of evening light exposure on the sleep of elderly women expressing sleep complaints. *Journal of Behavioral Medicine, 21*, 103–114.

Ford, D.E., & Kamerow, D.B. (1999). Epidemiologic study of sleep disturbances and psychiatric disorders: An opportunity for prevention? *Journal of the American Medical Association, 262*, 1479–1484.

Gillette, M.U. (1997). Cellular and biochemical mechanisms underlying circadian rhythms in vertebrates. *Current Opinion in Neurobiology, 7*, 797–804.

Gore, A.C. (1998). Circadian rhythms during aging. In C.V. Mobbs & P.R. Hof (Eds.), *Functional endocrinology of aging* (pp. 127–165). Basel: S. Karger.

Harper, D.G., Rheaume, Y., Manning, B., and Volicer, L. (1999). Light therapy in Alzheimer's disease. In L. Volicer & L. Bloom-Charette (Eds.), *Enhancing the quality of life in advanced dementia* (pp. 186–205). Philadelphia: Taylor & Francis.

Hauri, P.J. (1999). Consulting about insomnia: A method and some preliminary data. *Sleep, 16,* 344–350.

Hirshkowitz, M., Moore, C.A., Hamilton, C.R., Rando, K.C., & Karacan, I. (1992). Polysomnography of adults and elderly: Sleep architecture, respiration, and leg movements. *Journal of Clinical Neurophysiology, 9,* 56–63.

Jost, B.C., & Grossberg, G.T. (1996). The evolution of psychiatric symptoms in Alzheimer's disease: A natural history study. *Journal of the American Geriatrics Society, 44,* 1078–1081.

Little, J.T., Satlin, A., Sunderland, T., & Volicer, L. (1995). Sundown syndrome in severely demented patients with probable Alzheimer's disease. *Journal of Geriatric Psychiatry and Neurology, 8,* 103–106.

Montplaisir, J., Petit, D., Lorrain, D., Gauthier, S., & Nielsen, T. (1995). Sleep in Alzheimer's disease: Further considerations on the role of brainstem and forebrain cholinergic populations in sleep-wake mechanisms. *Sleep, 18,* 145–148.

Morin, C.M., Culbert, J.P., & Schwartz, S.M. (1994). Nonpharmacological interventions for insomnia: A meta-analysis of treatment efficacy. *American Journal of Psychiatry, 151,* 1172–1180.

Morita, Y., Uchida, K., & Okamoto, N. (1996). Melatonin rhythm of Alzheimer's patients. *Frontiers of Hormone Research, 21,* 180–185.

Prinz, P.N., Vitaliano, P.P., Vitiello, M.V., Bokan, J., Raskind, M., Peskind, E., & Gerber, C. (1982). Sleep, EEG and mental function changes in senile dementia of the Alzheimer's type. *Neurobiology of Aging, 3,* 361–370.

Rheaume, Y.L., Manning, B.C., Harper, D.G., & Volicer, L. (1998). Effect of light therapy upon disturbed behaviors in Alzheimer's patients. *American Journal of Alzheimer's Disease, 13,* 291–295.

Rodin, J., McAvay, G., & Timko, C. (1988). A longitudinal study of depressed mood and sleep disturbances in elderly adults. *Journal of Gerontology, 43,* 45–53.

Satlin, A., Volicer, L., Stopa, E.G., & Harper, D. (1995). Circadian locomotor activity and core-body temperature rhythms in Alzheimer's disease. *Neurobiology of Aging, 16,* 765–771.

Spielman, A.J., Saskin, P., & Thorpy, M.J. (1987). Treatment of chronic insomnia by restriction of time in bed. *Sleep, 10,* 45–56.

Swaab, D.F., Fliers, E., & Partiman, T.S. (1985). The suprachiasmatic nucleus of the human brain in relation to sex, age and senile dementia. *Brain Research, 342,* 37–44.

Van Someren, E.J.W., Kessler, A., Mirmiran, M., & Swaab, D.F. (1997). Indirect bright light improves circadian rest-activity rhythm disturbances in demented patients. *Biological Psychiatry, 41,* 955–963.

Van Someren, E.J.W., Mirmiran, M., & Swaab, D.F. (1993). Non-pharmacological treatment of sleep and wake disturbances in aging and Alzheimer's disease: Chronobiological perspectives. *Behavioural Brain Research, 57,* 235–253.

Ware, J.C., & Morin, C.M. (1997). Sleep in depression and anxiety. In M.R. Pressman & W.C. Orr (Eds.), *Understanding sleep: The evaluation and treatment of sleep disorders* (pp. 483–503). Washington, DC: American Psychological Association.

# 12

# Apathy and Agitation

Agitation and apathy denote a lack of psychological well-being. They are likely to occur as dementia worsens and as people experience functional and cognitive decline. People with dementia lose the ability to make sense of their environment, to filter the stimulation that comes their way, to handle the stress of what is happening to them, and to cope with what is going on around them. The inability to initiate meaningful activities that engage individuals with their environment is one of dementia's major effects (see Chapter 6). As a consequence, this inability may lead to apathy, agitation, or both.

> Mrs. Luke is a 75-year-old retired elementary schoolteacher who lives with her son and daughter-in-law, Larry and Laura, and their two children. Mrs. Luke is a widow of 10 years. She was diagnosed as having Alzheimer's disease 3 years ago. She lived alone until last year when, in anticipation of increasing needs for assistance as her disease progressed, her children strongly advised her to sell the family house and move in with Larry's family. Mrs. Luke has problems remembering recent events, such as having taken a shower the night before. She makes poor decisions about aspects of her personal care; for example, she might dress for the wrong season if Laura does not select her daily clothing. She can help Laura prepare meals but cannot begin to prepare a meal by herself (mild dementia).

Mrs. Luke has two other children and six grandchildren, all of whom reside in the area. Laura and Larry both work full-time, and their children, Lindsay and Linda, are in the 5th and 8th grades. Laura has always had a wonderful relationship with her mother-in-law, and the two women have enjoyed doing things together, especially cooking and sewing. Laura works near her home and comes home for lunch as often as she can to check on Mrs. Luke. Today, Laura came home for lunch and found Mrs. Luke staring at the wall. Laura is quite concerned about her mother-in-law.

## APATHY

Apathetic people appear passive, demonstrate inattention to the external environment (e.g., fixed staring or immobility), and act uninterested in what is happening around them. People with dementia who are not provided with a meaningful activity often sit motionless, stare into space with a vacant expression, and show indifference and emotional disengagement. Apathy is a symptom that is observed in 80% of community-dwelling outpatients. Apathy differs from dysphoria (sad mood) and depression, both of which cause people to appear withdrawn.

### APATHY AND DEPRESSION

Apathy and depression are not synonymous. People may be apathetic but not necessarily depressed. For example, when apathy was compared to depression using the Neuropsychiatric Inventory (Cummings et al., 1994), there was no significant correlation to connect the two (Levy et al., 1998). Furthermore, although the presence of apathy was modestly correlated with dysphoria, which commonly accompanies depression, brain blood flow differed greatly between the two. Apathy was associated with severe prefrontal and anterior temporal hypoperfusion, whereas dysphoria had no related blood flow variation (Craig, Cummings, & Fairbanks, 1996).

When Larry came home from work, Laura described what she had observed at lunch. She noted that unless someone engages Mrs. Luke in an activity or a conversation, Mrs. Luke is apathetic. They are sad to see this dear woman, who was so involved with people and was so proud of her homemaking skills, especially cooking and sewing, so disconnected. Both Laura and Larry agree that Mrs. Luke needs help, but they do not know what type or where they can find it. Laura decides to change her hours at work to part time and to come home for lunch every day. This way there will be someone for Mrs. Luke to be with, at least in the afternoon, because her grandchildren are involved with after-school activities and friends.

## APATHY AND ENGAGEMENT

Engagement is the opposite of apathy. Engagement involves attention to and participation in the external environment, such as involvement in a conversation or other meaningful activities. Engaged people with dementia are active and interested in what is going on around them. One goal of care is to help a person with dementia like Mrs. Luke become engaged. To do so, she must first be evaluated to determine the causes of her apathy. In general, when a new behavioral symptom appears, an assessment is conducted for causes such as an underlying medical problem or a drug side effect. If no medical problem or drug side effect is found, then one determines what aspects of the dementing process are causing the problem, because peripheral behavioral symptoms are expressions of more basic processes.

The dementing process causes functional impairment and possibly delusions/hallucinations and depression, which in turn lead to spatial disorientation, anxiety, dependence in activities of daily living, and inability to initiate and engage in meaningful activities. Mrs. Luke's apathy may be the result of her functional impairment, which precludes her from engaging in activities she once did well and liked. Furthermore, even though neuropsychiatric symptoms are distinct entities, a person may have more than one. Mrs. Luke's lack of engagement could result from both apathy and depression.

Laura realizes that Mrs. Luke no longer finds things to do on her own initiative. She has even become limited in what she is able to do with someone helping her. Mrs. Luke has become passive—just sitting for hours and hours. Laura and Larry know that Mrs. Luke needs to be connected with the world and to be stimulated by some activity. The Luke's next-door neighbor suggests that Laura think about "day care" for Mrs. Luke. Both Laura and Larry think of "day care" as a place where children go when parents work rather than a place where parents go when children work. The Lukes discover several adult day centers that specialize in providing activity programs for older people. They decide to try one.

After talking with staff at the day center, Larry decides Mrs. Luke will attend 3 days a week and arranges for her transportation to and from the center. Laura makes an unannounced visit to the center to check on her mother-in-law and finds Mrs. Luke happily socializing with another older woman. Seeing her mother-in-law engaged with another person makes Laura feel good about the day services decision.

Eventually, however, Laura notices that Mrs. Luke is restless when she gets home from the day center in the afternoon. One day, when she is not at the day center, Mrs. Luke paces back and forth between the kitchen and living room. She finally calms down when Laura sits with her and looks through a favorite cookbook with her and talks about the happy memories that she associates with each of the special recipes.

## AGITATION

When Mrs. Luke does not demonstrate apathy, she manifests agitation. In fact, it is common for individuals with dementia to have bouts of apathy followed by agitation. It is important to assess possible causes of agitation to direct care to its cause. Use the following guidelines in your assessment:

1. Eliminate the physical and medical causes of agitation.

- Has the person been ill or suffered a recent injury?
- Does the person feel any physical discomfort or pain?
- Does the person have any medical complications such as a urinary tract infection?
- Could a fall have occurred that injured the person?

2. Look for any aspect of the dementia that may be the underlying problem that contributes to the behavior.

- Depression
- Delusions or hallucinations
- Inability to initiate meaningful activity
- Spatial disorientation

3. Look for a pattern or trigger to the behavior.

- Does the behavior occur at any set time of day?
- Does the behavior occur after the person takes a certain drug?
- Does the behavior occur when the person is hungry?
- Does the behavior occur when the person is frustrated?
- Does the behavior occur when the person has been with a certain individual?

4. Look for events that could contribute to the behavior.

- When the problem was first noticed, were there any other changes in the way in which the person was acting at that time, such as a persisting change in mood?
- When the problem was first noticed, were there any significant changes in the person's home situation?

—Had the person or primary caregiver moved residences?

—Did anyone else move in or out of the house?

—Did anyone in the family die or become ill?

—Were there any changes in care arrangements such as starting or stopping day services?

- When the problem was first noticed, did the person start any new medications or were any drugs or dosages changed?

5. Look for immediate events that could directly cause the behavior (e.g., being in a difficult situation).

- Was the person asked to complete a task that was too complex?
- Did the person have a frustrating interaction with another individual?
- Was the person exposed to a chaotic or overstimulating environment?

6. Observe what happened.

- What were the undesirable behaviors of the person with dementia?
- Why did these behaviors occur?
- Try to answer the following:
  —What emotions did the person show?
  —Who else was present?
  —How did others respond?

7. Note the consequences of the behavior.

- What happened to the person with dementia?
- Who else was affected?
- What happened to others?

## PHYSICAL CAUSES

By uncovering the physical causes, it is easier to treat agitation before it escalates into assaultive or even violent behavior.

Laura concentrates on Mrs. Luke's physical needs that she may not be able to express. Because Mrs. Luke is served two meals at the day center, Laura thinks she is probably not hungry. The room is not cold or drafty, so Mrs. Luke is probably not uncomfortable because of the environment. Still, something triggers this behavior. Laura wonders whether Mrs. Luke is wandering restlessly because she is ill.

To be sure that there is no medical problem causing the symptoms, Laura arranges an afternoon appointment for Mrs. Luke to see her primary care provider. Mrs. Luke is unable to answer questions about her medical history. Laura provides an update of her mother-in-law's current condition, including the recent changes of apathy onset and the newly developed symptom of agitation. The nurse practitioner conducts an examination and finds no physical basis for Mrs. Luke's apathy and agitation. She gives Laura written instructions to prevent and manage agitation (see Tables 12.1 and 12.2).

Laura suspects that the change in Mrs. Luke's behavior could be caused by Lindsay and his friends. Now that Laura is home in the afternoons, Lindsay comes home after school, often with several of his friends. Although Mrs. Luke, a former elementary schoolteacher, loves children and always welcomed her grandchildren into her home, she can no longer cope with the stimulation of children's activities. Mrs. Luke no longer remembers her grandchildren's names. What used to be a joyful experience, watching her grandchildren play, is now a situation she cannot understand. Too much activity and noise now agitate Mrs. Luke.

**Table 12.1.   *General guidelines to prevent or minimize agitated behaviors in the person with dementia***

Make sure the person is physically comfortable. Assess and remediate all known physical needs of the person. Be sure the person is not too hot or cold, hungry or thirsty, tired, wet, overstimulated, or bored.

Stay calm and avoid showing frustration. It is important to look relaxed despite any upset feelings. An individual with dementia is able to pick up on the emotional content of another person, so caregivers need to be aware of how they say something, as well as what their body language and facial expressions are saying. They should smile as much as possible, use slow hand gestures, keep their body relaxed, and establish eye contact. People with dementia have lost their ability to process the meaning of another's frustration. If a caregiver exhibits frustration, therefore, people with dementia may easily become frustrated themselves.

Provide reassurance and emotional support. Speak slowly and clearly. People with dementia may not be able to acknowledge caregiver emotional support, but, nevertheless, they can recognize and appreciate supportive actions. Therefore, caregivers should smile genuinely, nod their heads in agreement, convey a helpful demeanor, and keep the tone and speed of their voices moderate and avoid yelling. They should be aware of the person's possible hearing loss and remember that dementia makes it harder to understand many words.

Make the environment calm and quiet and provide a sense of security. People with dementia can become agitated if their environment is overly stimulating, so it is important for them to avoid loud noises, places that are too busy, and too many people talking at once.

Ignore problematic behavior unless it is a safety concern. If the behavior is only a nuisance as opposed to a potential hazard, "live with it," no matter how annoying. If a person with dementia is having a loud but pleasant one-way conversation in response to a hallucination or to a person on television, so be it.

Know the person's level of orientation, but make the assessment without giving a "pop quiz," asking questions that are beyond the person's ability to answer.

*(continued)*

**Table 12.1.** — continued

People with dementia may be frustrated because they do not know who they are, where they are, or what day it is. A gentle reminder can relieve the frustration. Being forced to remember when they cannot, or having reality imposed on them, may only increase their frustration.

Meet people where they are. People with dementia can easily become frustrated if a task or request is too complex, yet adults should not be infantilized. People may feel upset if a task or request is too simple. Establish what they can do and understand, and meet them at that place.

Do not expect a person with dementia to adapt. Instead, change the environment as much as possible to accommodate the person. Avoid asking an individual with dementia to adapt to a new place or learn a new task.

Take a caregiver time-out. The person with dementia will quickly forget recent events. If what you are trying is not working, stop, leave, and then return and start fresh with a new approach. Time-outs also allow you to calm down if the situation has been particularly frustrating for you.

Learn and apply knowledge of the person's history, culture, and first language. People with dementia often live more in the past than in the present. Knowing who they were before their dementia began gives you both something positive to talk about. Knowing the person's culture can help the caregiver to understand the person's problematic behaviors and provide coping solutions. Dementia can lead to forgetting second languages. The language of origin also can be comforting when heard.

Do not argue with people with dementia. Avoid reasoning or trying to convince people with dementia of something because they have lost their cognitive abilities. They can become frustrated by not understanding or because they are talking to someone who is frustrated. Avoid conflicts instead of confronting people with dementia. Agree as often as possible. Avoid using the word "no." Even if people with dementia believe dead spouses are still alive (because they do not remember the death), do not try to convince them otherwise because reality orientation can lead to agitation, frustration, and anger. Besides, believing that a spouse is still alive can be comforting to them.

Reframe issues by putting things another way. Reframing is useful when people with dementia cannot understand a concept. Use single words that are familiar and nonthreatening. Be ready to try new words or phrases if those being used are not working.

Prevent or avoid situations that can invoke frustration, a precursor of agitation. Limit choices. Ask yes-or-no questions. Do not ask people with dementia to do more than they are capable of doing.

Avoid conversations in crowded or loud places. Someone with dementia can be easily startled. It is hard to focus on one conversation when many others are going on or to concentrate when startled.

Acknowledge what the person has said. Repeat key points and words to let the person with dementia know you heard him or her. Nod your head in agreement.

Rephrase upsetting statements. People with dementia may not recognize or understand the words that caregivers use or the words may be disturbing to them. Try to find simple and comforting terms. For example, the Bedford Geriatric Research, Education and Clinical Center's Adult Day Care Center is called the Veterans' Center. The hallways and gathering areas contain pictures of the participants in their service uniforms. It is their "club." Instead of quarreling about going to day services, veterans look forward to going to the club.

Agitation, an unpleasant state of excitement, is manifested by physical or vocal behaviors or both. Agitation can be caused by internal and/or external stimuli and is different from other negative states such as discomfort or resistiveness to care that occurs during an interaction with a caregiver. A person with dementia who is agitated appears restless. The Luke family learned that Mrs. Luke is able to cope with only a certain amount of stimulation. They adjusted their routines to provide what they considered to be the right amount of day services, socialization, and diversion without too much commotion. The family did not want to overwhelm Mrs. Luke, but they did not want her to revert to becoming apathetic either. Also, Lindsay was asked to stop bringing his friends home to play.

> Laura feels a little better knowing that there are tangible actions she can take to make things better for her mother-in-law. She teaches Lindsay and Linda some strategies to help avoid agitating their grandmother. The afternoons that Mrs. Luke does not go to the day center, Laura sits and does something relaxing with her mother-in-law. Going over the old cookbooks is Mrs. Luke's favorite activity. It is boring for Laura to do the same thing every day, but not for Mrs. Luke, the person to whom the activity is directed. So, Laura goes through the cookbook and talks about the same special memories day after day. Mrs. Luke is quite content, although she sometimes becomes sad and tearful when she hears about a favorite meal of her deceased husband's.

**Table 12.2.    General guidelines to manage agitated behaviors in the person with dementia**

Use distraction and redirection. If the person is getting upset, use short-term memory loss to the caregiver's advantage—the person with dementia may easily forget what caused the upset. Change the topic, take the person's attention off his or her immediate goal(s), gently guide the person away from what is upsetting, and help him or her to focus on something different. Find an outlet, such as taking a walk or playing a game.

Use visual cues. If people with dementia can still recognize their handwriting, sometimes gently showing them objects (e.g., calendars or notes in their own handwriting) can help.

Hit the "reset button": Stop. Immediately change the stimulus. If the person liked to play solitaire, give him or her a deck of cards and a quiet place to play.

Try a "loving deception." For example, use simulated presence therapy and take advantage of a well-liked and familiar voice. Say, for example, "Here's a telephone call for you" and place the handset on the person.

Respond to the emotion, not the behavior. The person may be frightened or anxious. Focus on feelings, not on facts. Listen to the body language and facial expressions of the person and provide reassurance.

Try a relaxing or diversional activity such as music or perhaps massage. Sit down with the person and use a treasured photo album to engage him or her in reminiscence therapy by looking at the pictures and recalling special memories.

About a month later, Laura received a call at work to come immediately to the day center. Mrs. Luke was out of control. She had hit another participant and the staff could not handle such an angry outburst. Laura had never seen her mother-in-law in such a negative state of excitement. Mrs. Luke cried and yelled at Laura, "Where did you put my husband? I want my husband! I want my husband! Get away from me! Go away! Where's my husband?"

## DEPRESSION

Although they are distinct conditions, there is a relationship between agitation and depression. Symptoms of depression in people with dementia include agitation, restlessness, repetitive vocalization, irritability, and combative behavior (see Chapter 3). When people with dementia are stressed, catastrophic behaviors may result because of untreated or undertreated depression (Hall & Buckwalter, 1987).

When Mrs. Luke asked where her husband was, another day center participant who had known Mr. Luke told her that her husband was dead. When Mrs. Luke started to cry and continued to ask about her husband, the other participant said, "I told you, he's dead!" That comment was what precipitated Mrs. Luke's hitting the woman. Unfortunately, the day center program staff had minimal training in caring for people with dementia, so they were not prepared to handle Mrs. Luke's repetitive requests for information and her angry outburst. Laura distracted Mrs. Luke by talking about the special foods she liked to prepare for Mr. Luke. She redirected Mrs. Luke to an activity. Laura gently takes Mrs. Luke's hand and looks into her eyes to gain her attention and says, "Yes, I know Dad [her name for Mr. Luke] well ... He loves to play cards." Laura then redirected Mrs. Luke by gently guiding her to the card table and giving her a deck of cards to "have them shuffled for Mr. Luke," a therapeutic deception. (See Table 12.2 for guidelines to manage agitation nonpharmacologically.)

After Laura brought her mother-in-law home, she tried to get her settled by using the tried-and-true strategy of the cookbook reminiscence. Unfortunately, Laura could not redirect Mrs. Luke to be calm. Mrs. Luke became angry with Laura and shouted, "Why are you doing this to me? Go away! Go away!" Then Mrs. Luke reached out to hit Laura. Laura was shocked.

When Larry came home for dinner, he found the children in the family room. His mother was crying in the living room, and Laura was crying in their bedroom. Laura sobbed to Larry about how guilty she feels for putting her mother-in-law in the day center and how upset she is that his mother is mad at her: "Maybe she has resented me for years and it's just coming out now."

Larry took his mother to the doctor's office the next day and met with the same nurse practitioner who had seen Mrs. Luke previously. The nurse practitioner makes the diagnosis of depression (see Chapter 3). Untreated depression coupled with the inability to initiate meaningful activities could make Mrs. Luke angry, which she expresses through her agitated behaviors. The nurse practitioner prescribes a low dose of an antidepressant (50 mg of sertraline [Zoloft]) each morning.

The nature of the principal problems facing individuals with a progressive dementia varies with their stage of dementia. In the early stages the main problem usually is the cognitive deficit that results in memory problems, spatial disorientation, and apraxia. Mrs. Luke had been suffering from apathy followed by agitation and then possibly from depression manifested by angry outbursts and mood swings. Mrs. Luke's symptoms could be a consequence of discomfort caused by a physical illness. If so, then correcting the underlying problem should alleviate the behavioral symptoms. If no reversible medical problem could be found, then Mrs. Luke would need to be carefully evaluated to determine which aspects of the dementing process are triggering the behavioral symptoms (see model of behavioral symptoms of dementia in the Introduction and Chapters 3, 4, 6, and 8). This evaluation is important because if any of the core aspects of Mrs. Luke's dementia caused her symptoms, those symptoms could be managed more effectively by treating their underlying processes.

## RATIONALE FOR THERAPEUTICS

Therapeutic interventions for symptoms of dementia must have a sound rationale based on reliable research data indicating that the intervention is effective. Agitation and apathy also are symptoms of other psychiatric disorders. Therapeutics developed for those psychiatric disorders, however, should not be applied to people with dementia unless there is evidence of their specificity for this condition. By basing caregiving activities on a model of psychological well-being, pragmatic approaches to medicinal and other therapies can be logically applied.

### MODEL OF PSYCHOLOGICAL WELL-BEING

Agitation and apathy are central concepts in a model of psychological well-being that is specific for people with dementia (Figure 12.1). This model depicts how the worsening of dementia over time restricts the range of emotions and people's capacity to express them. Individuals without dementia can express a variety of mood states that are positive or negative and active or passive, to constitute four quadrants of the ellipse shown in Figure 12.1. As dementia progresses, individuals lose their ability to cognitively process their mood states and to express their emotions verbally. Thus they resort to other, primarily nonverbal, means of communication.

An observation study of nursing facility residents with dementia who exhibited either agitation or withdrawn behavior showed that it is possible to recognize six indicators of emotional state and psychological well-being: happy, engaged, calm, sad, withdrawn, and agitated (Volicer, Hurley, & Camberg, 1999). These indicators can be seen as opposite poles of three continua that can be measured empirically. The first continuum ranges from happy to sad and is expressed through an individual's facial expression. The second continuum ranges from calm to agitated and is expressed by the individual's body movements and vocalization. The third continuum ranges from engaged to apathetic and is expressed by the degree of the individual's involvement with the environment.

## MEDICATIONS

A low-dose antidepressant was prescribed for Mrs. Luke because the nurse practitioner believed that her angry outbursts were the outcome of untreated depression. There is no medication to treat agitation specifically. There are

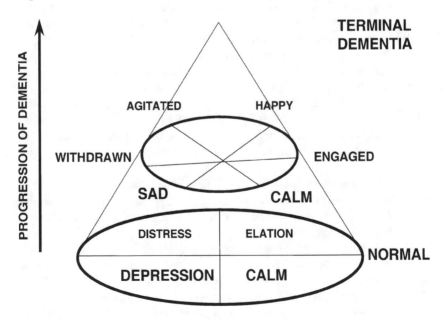

Figure 12.1. Model of psychological well-being for people with dementia.

many reasons why a person with dementia may be agitated, and interventions should be directed to the underlying cause. Two rules are useful:

1. Do not treat agitation as a separate problem that is unrelated to the basic dementing process that has produced the core and secondary symptoms.
2. Remember that undesirable side effects of antipsychotic and antianxiety medications can persist longer than the behaviors that the drugs were used to treat.

If unpleasant delusions or hallucinations were the source of Mrs. Luke's agitation, then a low-dose antipsychotic medication would be considered to treat the underlying cause of agitation.

The rational use of medications as interventions to manage challenging behaviors is complex. It may be tempting to try an antipsychotic medication to treat agitation, but drugs prescribed strictly for sedating purposes are no more than chemical restraints and should not be used. Yet, people who are agitated are uncomfortable, and they may act in ways that may be harmful to themselves and others. Therefore, if a medication can alleviate troublesome symptoms and provide comfort for the person, then the drug should be tried. Medications in this case, however, should not be the first line of intervention. Instead, they should be considered after nonpharmacological strategies, including environmental changes, fail.

Because no medication treats agitation directly, only a medication to treat its specific underlying cause should be initiated. Sensible medication requires both the art and science of knowledgeable drug use. The science deals with the pharmacokinetics and pharmacodynamics of medications. The art of prescribing medications for the older adult with dementia is dependent on providers' ability to conduct a skillful and comprehensive assessment and identify the correct drug, dose, frequency, time, and route of administration. The provider must judge the drug's effectiveness based on desired and undesired effects and plan drug holidays to evaluate the continued need for the drug. General rules of medication for agitated behaviors are as follows:

1. Conduct a detailed assessment to identify all possible causes of agitation. Only when nonpharmacological strategies have been given a thorough trial or if medications are the only therapeutic treatment (e.g., delusions/hallucinations) should medications be considered.
2. Because there is no medication to treat agitation directly, caregivers should direct pharmacological treatment to the core or primary symptom(s) that may be the cause of the agitated behaviors.
3. Before medication is added to a care plan, review all existing medications and dosages for their intended and actual effects to avoid duplication, side effects, or interactions.

4.  Use interdisciplinary care planning to establish the desired treatment goal with measurable outcome(s) by a specific time.

## CAREGIVERS

Caregivers control the environment. The key is to apply the right amount of stimulation—to promote pleasure and prevent apathy without inciting agitation. Because Mrs. Luke is no longer able to initiate meaningful activities for herself, Laura, Larry, and the day center staff should identify appropriate activities for Mrs. Luke and help her become engaged with them. They also should assess the causes and management of overstimulation (e.g., the boys playing at home, too many visitors, the television set).

Caregiving strategies involve the whole family, so specific education for each member must be provided. Mrs. Luke might not be able to remember her friends' names or those of her grandchildren, but this does not mean that she has no need for socialization. Although Mrs. Luke may not be able to initiate a social interaction, she still has a need to interact with others. Mrs. Luke's grandchildren must be taught how to be with their grandmother and how to interact with her without wearing her out. Visits from family and friends must be spaced rather than everyone visiting at the same time. Not all of the children and grandchildren should visit at the same time. Television programs and their effects on Mrs. Luke need to be monitored. She may get upset easily because of what she sees or hears on television, or she may no longer understand the box that has people in it and that emits so much noise.

Although Mrs. Luke continued to become more forgetful, things were all right for 6 months. Then, Mrs. Luke fell. Laura found her lying on the living room floor and called an ambulance to take her to the emergency room. Mrs. Luke broke her hip. She had surgery and her hip healed well, but her dementia worsened markedly while she recuperated in the hospital. Unfortunately, Mrs. Luke had to be restrained to keep her in bed and to prevent her from pulling out the intravenous tubing. Mrs. Luke became even more confused and agitated.

When acute care was no longer necessary, Mrs. Luke was transferred to a rehabilitation facility, where she received physical therapy and walked with staff assistance. The goal of care was for Mrs. Luke to walk without assistance so that she could return home, but Mrs. Luke did not learn to walk alone. She could not go home. Mrs. Luke was transferred again, this time to a long-term care facility.

Unfortunately, Mrs. Luke did not understand where she was and could not interact with the other residents. She spent most of the day staring vacantly. She also banged on her bedside rail or chair and yelled for help or demanded to go home. No physical causes that might precipitate these behaviors were identified. Laura and Larry were alarmed and saddened by these changes. When the family visited, they were able to engage Mrs. Luke when she was apathetic and to stop her agitation when she called out for help. The physical therapist helping Mrs. Luke ambulate also was able to have a somewhat interactive conversation with Mrs. Luke, but, when left to her own devices, Mrs. Luke had no contact with the world around her.

Mrs. Luke alternated between periods of agitation and apathy. Agitation is uncomfortable for the people who have it. Vocalizations that communicate their discomfort can actually worsen the condition. Because loud, negative vocalizations are disruptive to other residents and caregivers, agitation manifested by vocalization receives prompt attention. No one wants to hear another person hollering constantly that he or she wants to go home.

Apathy is not bothersome for other residents or disruptive to caregivers. Because apathetic people do not cry out or display intensive motor activity, their condition may go unnoticed. People with dementia who cannot express themselves verbally often let their behaviors communicate how they are feeling. People with apathy may "suffer in silence" unless their caregivers are sensitive to this symptom and take action.

## SIMULATED PRESENCE THERAPY

Except for her dementia and healing hip fracture, Mrs. Luke was a physically healthy woman who actively participated in visits from her family, and appeared distressed when they were not present. During their visits, the conversation focused on special family experiences. Staffing did not provide the one-to-one interaction that Mrs. Luke required. The recreation therapist suggested trying simulated presence therapy as an intervention.

Simulated presence therapy (SPT) uses selected memories to manage challenging behaviors. It is helpful for long-term care facility residents who have dementia (Woods & Ashley, 1995). Residents' best-loved experiences are selected from their long-term memories and audiotaped by a family member or staff member. The SPT technique records statements and questions related to the resident's experiences in the context of a normal, spontaneous conversation, much like an interview. The resulting one-sided, personalized conversational audiotape is played for a resident using a headset and an autoreverse tape player. Because of their dementia, residents have recent memory defects, and audiotaped messages can be played repeatedly and still be perceived as a fresh conversation each time.

In a large multicenter study involving 54 subjects, SPT was compared with a neutral recording (newspaper reading) and usual care (Camberg et al., 1999). According to nursing staff reports, SPT improved agitated behavior 75% more often than when the neutral recording was used and 35% more often than when usual care was provided. SPT also improved withdrawn behavior three times more often than did the neutral tape and 80% more often than did usual care. Independent observers found that study subjects were more likely to display a happy facial expression when they received SPT or personal attention.

> Larry made an SPT tape recording. Mrs. Luke responded to each repetition of the tape as if it were a new conversation. She nodded her head in agreement, smiled, and looked relaxed. Her psychological well-being improved dramatically with the use of SPT. The long-term care staff also felt emotional relief because Mrs. Luke actually looked happy and there was something tangible that they could do when she presented with a vacant facial expression.

> The staff noticed that Mrs. Luke began to become agitated, for no apparent reason, in the late afternoon. They tried SPT as a routine diversion between her afternoon snack and dinner. Using the tape prevented Mrs. Luke from becoming agitated. Laura and Larry were relieved when the staff reported that Mrs. Luke was less agitated when they were not able to be with her in person. Larry, especially, feels empowered to improve his mother's quality of life because many of the previous caregiving activities have been performed by Laura. He is actually making a tangible contribution to his mother's well-being!

## SUNDOWN SYNDROME

Mrs. Luke was experiencing what some caregivers refer to as "sundowning" or "sundown syndrome." Sundowning is best defined as "the appearance or exacerbation of behavioral disturbances associated with the afternoon and/or evening hours" (Little, Satlin, Sunderland, & Volicer, 1995, p. 103). This syndrome is a poorly defined entity. Some investigators even question its existence because some patients are more agitated in the morning, some are more agitated in the afternoon and evening, and some are equally agitated throughout the day (Bliwise, Carroll, Lee, Nekich, & Dement, 1993; Cohen-Mansfield et al., 1989). Whether or not it is a distinct clinical entity, sundown syndrome appears to be a behavioral characteristic of at least some individuals with dementia. Sundowning has been ascribed to environmental influences such as change of shift (Exum, Phelps, Nabers, & Osborne, 1993) or to attempts of confused individuals to leave a dementia care unit because they "want to go home from work." Sundowning may be related to disturbances in circadian rhythm (described in Chapter 11), which includes a condition that is similar to jet lag. Light therapy is used to treat insomnia caused by a circadian rhythm disturbance, and it also may be effective in reducing sundown syndrome. Furthermore, an experience earlier in the day may cause agitation later in the day or at night. Or, if the person receives a hypnotic to promote nighttime sleep, then the sedative effect could last until the afternoon, resulting in agitation when the hypnotic effects abate.

## SUPPORT FOR FAMILY CAREGIVERS

Despite continuing the rehabilitation efforts, Mrs. Luke did not regain her ability to walk. She also became incontinent. Her care was too difficult for her family to manage at home, so Laura and Larry, with deep regret, made the decision for Mrs. Luke to remain in long-term care. Mrs. Luke was transferred to a "life-long care" facility in another part of the hospital. This decision was particularly hard on Laura, who feels that she has failed her mother-in-law. Laura had been feeling guilty ever since Mrs. Luke's angry outburst at her, and "putting her in the home" only exacerbated the guilt. Mrs. Luke's physical and mental conditions worsened from the combination of the new environment and new staff plus her progressing dementia. In addition, Mrs. Luke developed sleeping problems. She would wake several times during the night and repeatedly call out for her husband, saying she wanted to go home. Mrs. Luke needs medication to treat her condition, and Laura needs to work through her feelings of guilt.

Mrs. Luke had previously received sertraline to treat depression, which is believed to be the cause of her angry outbursts in the day center. When she was admitted to acute care for her fractured hip, Mrs. Luke's sertraline was not ordered, and her depression recurred. The interdisciplinary team in the long-term unit revised her care plan and restarted sertraline. This plan was working to make Mrs. Luke more comfortable, but Laura felt guiltier than ever. First, she believed that she was responsible for not telling the long-term unit staff that she had been giving Mrs. Luke a daily medication for depression. She also felt conflicted about "drugging" her mother-in-law. The social worker who worked with the Luke family to transfer Mrs. Luke to her current unit had previously encouraged Laura to join a support group. Finally, Laura agreed to attend a support group meeting to get help in working through her guilt.

Many caregivers believe that they have failed the person in their care and have guilty feelings about it. Laura needed to learn and internalize the fact that despite the finest caregiving possible, dementia worsens. Laura was similar to many other good caregivers, feeling that she let her mother-in-law down. Laura could not prevent the dementia from worsening. Mrs. Luke probably had not resented Laura, and by the time of the angry outbursts, Mrs. Luke no longer had the capacity to resent anyone.

> Laura joined a support group of adult children of people with dementia. It took a while, but Laura eventually was able to talk about her feelings of guilt. After 5 months, Mrs. Luke developed pneumonia and died. The Luke family grieved but had no regrets about their care for Mrs. Luke because they did everything they could do. The dementia caused terrible symptoms that were uncomfortable for Mrs. Luke and distressing for all who loved and cared for her.

Coping with dementia is challenging, not just for the person with dementia but also for his or her family, caregivers, and loved ones. They need help to alleviate any sense of failure or guilt that they may be feeling. Families, caregivers, and loved ones are people who deserve help, concern, and respect. They should be encouraged and helped to express any negative emotions regarding their own and their loved ones' experiences with the person with dementia. Grief adjustment is complex and requires considerable support and guidance from others (Rheaume & Brown, 1998). The professional caregiver's role is to help families cope by fostering a sense of self-respect and pride in their own accomplishments, in the care of their loved one, and in their own survival during the progression of their loved one's dementia (Brown, Lyons, & Sellers, 1988).

## REFERENCES

Bliwise, D.L., Carroll, J.S., Lee, K.A., Nekich, J.C., & Dement, W.C. (1993). Sleep and sundowning in nursing home residents with dementia. *Psychiatry Research, 48,* 277–292.

Brown, J., Lyon, P.C., & Sellers, T.D. (1988). Caring for the family caregivers. In L. Volicer, K.J. Fabiszewski, Y.L. Rheaume, & K.E. Lasch (Eds.), *Clinical management of Alzheimer's disease* (pp. 29–41). Rockville, MD: Aspen Publishers.

Camberg, L., Woods, P., Ooi, W.L., Hurley, A., Volicer, L., Ashley, J., Odenheimer, G., & McIntyre, K. (1999). Evaluation of simulated presence: A personalized approach to enhance well-being in persons with Alzheimer's disease. *Journal of the American Geriatrics Society, 47*(4), 446–452.

Cohen-Mansfield, J., Watson, V., Meade, W., Gordon, M., Leatherman, J., & Emor, C. (1989). Does sundowning occur in residents of an Alzheimer's unit? *International Journal of Geriatric Psychiatry, 4,* 293–298.

Craig, A.H., Cummings, J.L., & Fairbanks, L. (1996). Cerebral blood flow correlates of apathy in Alzheimer disease. *Archives of Neurology, 53,* 1116–1120.

Cummings, J.L., Mega, M., Gray, K., Thompson, S.R., Carusi, D.A., & Gornbein, J. (1994). Comprehensive assessment of psychopathology in dementia. *Neurology, 44,* 2308–2314.

Exum, M.E., Phelps, B.J., Nabers, K.E., & Osborne, J.G. (1993). Sundown syndrome: Is it reflected in the use of PRN medications for nursing home residents? *Gerontologist, 33,* 756–761.

Hall, G.R., & Buckwalter, K.C. (1987). Progressively lowered stress threshold: A conceptual model for care of adults with Alzheimer's disease. *Archives of Psychiatric Nursing, 1,* 399–406.

Levy, M.L., Cummings, J.L., Fairbanks, L.A., Masterman, D., Miller, B.L., Craig, A.H., Paulsen, J.S., & Litvan, I. (1998). Apathy is not a depression. *Journal of Neuropsychiatry, 10,* 314–319.

Little, J.T., Satlin, A., Sunderland, T., & Volicer, L. (1995). Sundown syndrome in severely demented patients with probable Alzheimer's disease. *Journal of Geriatric Psychiatry and Neurology, 8,* 103–106.

Rheaume, E.L., & Brown, J. (1998). Complexities of the grieving process in spouses of patients with Alzheimer's disease. In L. Volicer & A. Hurley (Eds.), *Hospice care for patients with advanced progressive dementia* (pp. 189–204). New York: Springer.

Volicer, L., Hurley, A., & Camberg, L. (1999). A model of psychological well being in advanced dementia. *Journal of Mental Health and Aging, 5,* 83–94.

Woods, P., & Ashley, J. (1995). Simulated presence therapy: Using selected memories to manage problem behaviors in Alzheimer's disease. *Geriatric Nursing, 16*(1), 9–14.

# 13

# Elopement and Interference with Others

One fear expressed by caregivers of people with dementia is that the person under their care will elope (wander away) and become lost or injured or die. Elopement is a potential problem in all settings where individuals with dementia reside. A combination of care-recipient and environmental factors determines the risk for elopement and suggests individualized preventive strategies and early intervention programs. Prevention of elopement without needless restriction presents a challenge because caregivers need to anticipate how, when, and why people with dementia might leave their safe environment unattended.

Mrs. Myrna Minkiezich is a 79-year-old Russian who emigrated to a suburb of a large East Coast city 5 years ago. She lives with her granddaughter, Minska, who defected from the former Soviet Union to join an American ballet company. Life had been hard in Russia. Mrs. Minkiezich's husband disappeared, and her three sons died in the conflict in Afghanistan, leaving her alone. Mrs. Minkiezich was raised as an Orthodox Jew but had to practice her religion clandestinely until coming to the United States. Mrs. Minkiezich is very happy being able to practice her religion openly and go to temple. Her religion is very important to her. Mrs. Minkiezich's only living blood relative is Minska, who made the arrangements for her grandmother to move in with her family, which includes her husband and two daughters. Mrs. Minkiezich does not speak English, and she stays at home except for attending temple.

Mrs. Minkiezich has mild Alzheimer's disease that had been difficult to diagnose because of the language barrier. It has been easy for Minska to take care of Mrs. Minkiezich because Minska is ebullient and outgoing, with an easygoing and happy personality. Mrs. Minkiezich requires increasing assistance with getting dressed, oversight to make sure she eats, and help finding something to do during the day. One afternoon, Minska comes home from ballet practice to find her home empty. Her grandmother is gone.

## ELOPEMENT

The exact prevalence of elopement in people with dementia is unknown. Wandering (presumably unattended and not "permitted" by caregivers) occurs in up to 65% of nursing facility residents and dementia clinic patients and 36% of people with dementia living in the community (Logsdon et al., 1998). When a person with dementia is missing for hours, becomes injured, or dies, the issue of elopement receives much attention. The tragic death of a missing person is reported in the lay press and discussed in caregiver support groups, and it raises the consciousness of the community. The extent of elopement from the home, congregate housing, assisted living, or licensed long-term care facilities is not known. One reason for not knowing the prevalence of elopement is that several terms are used to describe the ambulating behaviors of people with dementia. These terms are poorly and inconsistently defined. When used in the context of a particular situation, often they describe a "nuisance" behavior for caregivers or residents without dementia, instead of a life-threatening behavior for the person with dementia.

### WANDERING BEHAVIORS

Wandering is the catchall term used in the literature to label "inappropriate ambulation" of people with dementia. What is inappropriate to the caregiver may seem appropriate to the person with dementia. An individual might be searching for something, attempting to fulfill unmet needs, "killing time," escaping a threatening situation, reacting to reminders of departure near an exit, or carrying out a predementia lifestyle function.

Wandering commonly describes the ambulating behavior of a person with dementia when that person walks away from one area or walks into an area "without permission." The adjective definition of wandering is characterized by aimless, slow, or pointless movements. The first noun definition is a going about from place to place, and the second noun definition is movement away from the proper, normal, or usual course or place. Among professional caregivers, the term *wandering* is used with an implicit understanding that it is a problematic behavior of the person with dementia. That general term, however, is too imprecise to guide interventions. Instead of "wandering," a specific description such as "walking repeatedly into others' rooms" is more useful to analyze these behaviors (Strumpf, Robinson, Wagner, & Evans, 1998).

Four questions that need to be posed are

1. What are the defining characteristics of problematic ambulation given that people with dementia have decreased cognitive capacity but may not have physical problems that interfere with their physical capacity to ambulate?
2. How can safe exercise be provided?
3. Is all unaccompanied ambulation problematic?
4. If unaccompanied ambulation is a problem, then who has the problem?

People with dementia do not differ from individuals without dementia in needing to move about, to change location, to exercise, to feel unconfined, and to work off pent-up energy. There are many behaviors that alone are not harmful to the person with dementia or to others. They are labeled as problematic, however, because they are bothersome and they require extra time and energy from an already-depleted caregiver.

In a residential setting, the term *wandering* may be used when the person with dementia enters the room of another resident. From the perspective of the resident whose room is entered without permission, however, the issue is invasion of privacy and, perhaps, loss of personal articles if the wanderer rummages through a closet or chest of drawers and takes something. Because of wandering aimlessly into another's room and seeing an open (and inviting) closet, the person with dementia can unwittingly interfere with other residents.

## PACING

Another term used to describe unaccompanied ambulating behavior in individuals with dementia is *pacing*. Pacing behaviors are characterized by repetitively walking back and forth as if following a rhythm or pattern. Pacing often occurs with speed and a sense of urgency and may seem to represent hyperactivity or restlessness. Pacing is problematic for the person with dementia when it occupies so much waking time that the person becomes overtired and experiences the consequences of fatigue. If pacing interferes with sitting down to eat or requires more calories than the person's daily intake provides, and thus poses a risk of malnutrition, or if it causes foot problems such as blisters, then caregivers should intervene to limit it. Otherwise, pacing is not problematic and the environment should be adapted to allow safe and controlled pacing that does not interfere with others. Often, people with dementia do not get enough exercise, so controlled pacing may, in fact, be a desirable physical activity.

Minska receives a call from her rabbi that Mrs. Minkiezich is sitting in the temple by herself. Mrs. Minkiezich cannot get dressed without Minska laying out her clothes and never goes to temple alone. Minska is relieved that Mrs. Minkiezich is "found," but she is perplexed about how Mrs. Minkiezich dressed by herself and went out alone. Minska goes to the temple. She finds her grandmother in her winter coat, although it is May. Otherwise, her grandmother looks fine.

The rabbi knows that Mrs. Minkiezich has a memory impairment and is confused. He is concerned that she might elope from Minska's home again, only to go to another place, with dire consequences. Because there are many elderly members of the temple who have physical and mental frailties, the rabbi is aware of many community programs. He suggests to Minska that she place some type of identification on Mrs. Minkiezich's clothing so she can be identified if she becomes lost.

Minska is upset about having to put labels in her grandmother's clothing. Identification and labeling reminds her too much of labeling Jews and other "undesirables" during the Holocaust. She dislikes the idea of putting a label on her grandmother the way in which Jews had to wear a yellow star of David on their clothing. The thought of her grandmother wearing an identification bracelet is too closely linked to the men and women in concentration camps whose forearms were tattooed with identification numbers. However, the rabbi convinces Minska that something must be done to help her grandmother be found if she wanders.

The issue of labeling clothing and related items is a classic example of the need to provide for safety while ensuring dignity (i.e., without infantilizing an adult). Two ways to circumvent this problem are to

- Sew labels that include the name of the individual and the name of the person to call if the person is found, into the inside lining of outerwear and in place of the commercial label on undergarments.
- Purchase a customized piece of jewelry (e.g., charm bracelet, watchband, chain with medallion) with an engraving of the individual's name and

whom to call if the person is found. Present this jewelry to the person as a special present and encourage the person to wear it.

## EXPLANATORY MODEL

The explanatory model places the term *elopement* at the center (Figure 13.1), and it illustrates how underlying causes and the presence of precipitants can change harmless wandering into elopement. For example, a person with dementia who does not have the ability to initiate meaningful activities sees the front door, which is unlocked and in his or her wandering path (easy exit), and the coat rack with coats and hats (reminder about leaving), and may leave unattended. Many potential negative outcomes (consequences) may result from elopement.

The model is activated by the urge to walk, which leads to pacing or wandering, both of which have advantages for the person with dementia. Walking preserves independence and prevents the consequences of immobility, such as general deconditioning, muscle weakness, stiffness, stasis, and orthostatic hypotension. Immobility also increases the risk of urinary tract infections and pneumonia (Volicer, Brandeis, & Hurley, 1998). In addition, people with dementia who are unable to ambulate are at risk for developing pressure ulcers. Walking may be one of the few activities that people with dementia can pursue on their own, and it should be encouraged. The disadvantages of walking occur when the unsupervised or nondirected individual interferes with others or elopes.

People with dementia can "shadow" a caregiver and persistently follow that person. For example, a spouse caregiver in the home setting may be followed all over the house, even into the bathroom. In a residential setting, a person with dementia may enjoy walking with another resident, but one who may not want to be accompanied. Thus, the ostensibly nonbothersome activity of a person with dementia—walking—can be quite bothersome to others under certain circumstances and interfere with other residents.

Many factors contribute to turn the safe and "happy wanderer" into the person who has eloped. A number of causes and precipitants are listed in Figure 13.1, and other conditions can exacerbate the problem. Not being able to terminate, or shift, a behavior once initiated (graphomotor perseveration) perpetuates the behavior. It is an indicator of the central nervous system pathology that is present in people with dementia (Ryan et al., 1995), and it may be one cause of elopement. Once the person has started to walk, then wander, and he or she cannot stop, elopement occurs—the person cannot self-correct. The problem may be exacerbated if the person has mobility or gait problems or becomes fearful when walking into an uncomfortable environ-

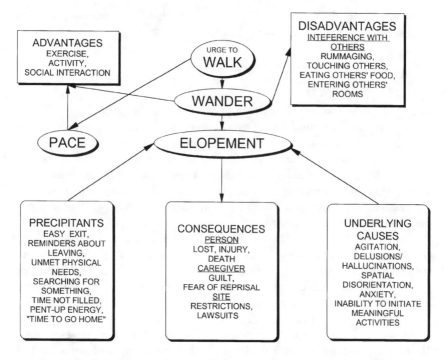

*Figure 13.1.    Explanatory model of elopement.*

ment. Most people with dementia who are lost do not have the capacity to ask for help. Searching for people with dementia is difficult because they no longer respond to their names. Thus, rescuers may be only a few feet away from individuals, yet not locate them.

Nursing facility residents who wander are at increased risk for injury because they are vulnerable to aggression from other residents on whose privacy they infringe. Elopement inside a building may put the person into unsafe areas such as stairwells, storage closets, or hazardous equipment areas. Outside elopement risks include exposure to the elements, being in traffic, getting lost, and, if not found, ultimately getting injured and even dying.

## THERAPEUTIC GOALS AND INTERVENTIONS

The primary caregiver goal is to prevent elopement and interference with other residents by providing safe outlets for the urge to walk. Successful management of primary and secondary dementia symptoms and precipitants to elopement is the second line of prevention. Treatment of all underlying causes of challenging behaviors should begin with a comprehensive assessment to identify the potential causes so that interventions can be directed to the root cause of the behavior. The guiding principle is that successful management requires a step-by-step analysis of the context, content, origins, and frequency of the behavior, its effects on others, and its consequences for the person with dementia (Alessi, 1991).

Accommodating the person's need to walk by promoting safe wandering and controlled pacing is beneficial because it provides the positive aspects of an exercise program, maintains mobility, and prevents deconditioning. Walking is a positive activity, and forms of independent walking, with proper safeguards, should be encouraged by caregivers for as long as possible during the progressive stages of dementia.

Interventions to prevent elopement should be directed to avert unsafe wandering, remove precipitants of elopement, and treat its underlying causes. Unsafe wandering may be altered by addressing specific etiological factors. Community-dwelling people with dementia who are cognitively impaired and behaviorally disturbed, who often sit alone, or who experience a high level of anxiety and depressive symptoms are more likely to wander (Logsdon et al., 1998). A darkened or unfamiliar environment, boredom, stress, tension, anxiety, lack of control, lack of exercise, and nocturnal delirium (which may be associated with the loss of spatial relationships in the dark) are factors that are related to wandering (Matteson & Linton, 1996).

## PERSON-FOCUSED PREVENTION OF ELOPEMENT

### Removal of the Precipitants of Elopement

The person with dementia who has nothing else to do and walks over to a well-marked and unlocked door may leave home or a unit unattended. If the person was involved with a meaningful activity or did not have easy access to an exit, then elopement would have been prevented. A coat hanging by the door or car keys lying on a table may be symbols that have long been associated with leaving and become stimuli for elopement. Being uncomfortable, too hot or cold, hungry, or thirsty may cause a person to seek relief from unpleasant symptoms by eloping. Routines from the person's predementia lifestyle may precipitate elopement by causing the desire to attend to a need, to go to work, or to be home for the children.

### Treatment of Underlying Causes Related to Dementing Illness

The underlying causes of elopement (Figure 13.1) can be uncomfortable for the person and therefore can be precipitants of elopement. Chapters 4, 6–8, and 12 describe interventions to manage delusions/hallucinations, the inability to initiate meaningful activities, anxiety, spatial disorientation, and agitation. Some manifestations of the underlying causes or precipitants of elopement can direct interventions to prevent it.

## Strategies Based on Knowledge of the Individual

A detailed assessment of the person's usual routine, including activity propensity, sleep–wake habits, and predementia lifestyle, should be made to individualize preventive interventions for elopement. For example, at a long-term care site, one man became very anxious around 4:00 P.M. He believed it was time to go home from work and would attempt to leave the unit. To prevent exiting attempts that could escalate into agitated behaviors, the staff helped him with his briefcase as he said his goodbyes to everyone. The telephone would ring (prearranged by staff) and he would be told that his bus was late and would pick him up after 6:00 P.M. He would take a short nap and wake up ready for dinner, forgetting that he had to go home (Simard, 1999).

The individual's type of wandering and potential elopement behavior determines the intervention (Warner, 1998). For example,

- "In search of" may be a quest to find something familiar, such as a childhood home, food, the bathroom, or a place to hide something.
- "To escape" may mean flight from a threat, such as a disturbing television show or to evade perceived mistreatment, or to get out of a frightening task, such as bathing.
- "With a purpose" may be an attempt to fulfill previous lifestyle responsibilities such as caring for children.
- "Aimless meandering" may result from having nothing else to do.

## ENVIRONMENT-FOCUSED INTERVENTIONS TO PREVENT ELOPEMENT

Indoor wandering is the safest type of wandering (Warner, 1998). Safe and simple wandering paths should be created in the environment, which should be adapted to be therapeutic for people with dementia.

## Environmental Modification

As the first-line optimal prevention, the physical environment in personal dwellings and long-term care units should exempt the exit door from the wandering path. If doing so is not possible, then visual barriers such as a cloth or blind to camouflage the door may control exiting (Dickinson, McLain-Kark, & Marshall-Baker, 1995). Spatial disorientation, whereby people misinterpret visual stimuli and respond to a two-dimensional pattern as if it were a three-dimensional object, can be used to limit wandering and elopement (Hewawasam, 1996). A stop sign on an exit door and an "off limits" sign by a fence are environmental cues that help to reduce attempts to exit (Matteson & Linton, 1996). A Dutch door, in which the top section, bottom section, or both sections may be opened or closed, allows controlled or free access to events beyond the door.

Minska develops elopement prevention strategies based on her grand-mother's lifestyle. Minska initiates the custom of having a picture taken of her grandmother during her birthday month so there will always be copies of recent pictures in case Mrs. Minkiezich elopes and outside help is needed. Minska orders labels that say, "If you find me alone, please call ..." and sews them into her grandmother's clothes. Mrs. Minkiezich loves the charm bracelet (with her name and address and the statement "If you find me alone, please call ...") given to her by her grandchildren, and she wears it every day. Minska locks Mrs. Minkiezich's bedroom closet that contains all of her clothes and places choices for the day on a small clothing rack. Minska realizes that she can no longer leave her grandmother unattended. The rabbi agrees with Minska's idea of having her grandmother go to temple each day to do "volunteer work," an alter-native to attending a day center.

The caregiving environment should be proactive to prevent elopement by meeting a person's needs for wandering. Because walking is a good activity that meets both the physical and social needs of people with dementia, it should be incorporated into care plans. In addition to those benefits, a walk-ing program also decreases aggression (Holmberg, 1997a), and it can be staffed by volunteers (Holmberg, 1997b), thus making it cost-effective.

## Devices

Although devices should not be the mainstay of prevention, there is a place for their rational use to limit wandering and prevent elopement. The use of three perimeter stages has been suggested (Warner, 1998):

- Stage 1 prevents access to areas of danger and elopement with door and window alarms and locks.
- Stage 2 allows limited wandering in certain areas by using door and win-dow alarms and locks, motion detectors with remote chimes, night-lights, Dutch doors, surveillance cameras, and intercom systems.
- Stage 3 prevents falls and notifies the caregiver of attempts to get out of bed or to get up from a chair. It uses a pull-tab alarm, a pressure-sensitive floor mat with an alarm, a monitor or surveillance camera, pressure-release chair or bed mats and alarms, and distance-monitoring devices and alarms.

Noise alarms or automatic door closing mechanisms have a negative side because they can be frightening, offensive, or stressful. The Jewish Home and Hospital Center in the Bronx, New York, addressed this issue in a special care unit by using a working dog. The dog was trained much like a seeing-eye dog except that instead of being assigned to one person, the dog watched the exit. When a resident attempted to leave, the dog guided the person back to the living room.

It has been several years since Minska's children were toddlers, but she remembers how she had to safety-proof her home. With the help of her husband and children, Minska surveys the house and decides where they should place devices to prevent her grandmother from eloping and to warn them, day and night, when she attempts to go outside. They put door latches high up and out of sight on the outside doors and decide to invest in a comprehensive alarm system, both for Mrs. Minkiezich's safety and to protect their home. The alarm company and the police are alerted to the fact that a person with cognitive impairment lives in the home. Minska feels confident about her grandmother's safety during the day, but she worries that she might get up in the middle of the night. She also worries that Mrs. Minkiezich will find the door latch and open it. To allay her fears, Minska buys a pressure-sensitive floor mat with a remote chime that rings in Minska's bedroom when Mrs. Minkiezich steps on the floor beside her bed. Once her grandmother goes to bed for the night, Minska activates the sensor.

## ESTABLISHMENT OF AN EARLY INTERVENTION PROGRAM

When a person has eloped, prompt discovery of the missing person usually means fewer negative consequences. Before someone begins to wander, the person should be registered with both the Alzheimer's Association Safe Return Program and the Medic Alert Program (Warner, 1998). Safe Return helps to find and return its members and helps guide the family through the ordeal (Silverstein & Flaherty, 1996).

Several other devices can help caregivers. The Alzheimer's Association brochure, *Products and Resources: A Listing of Items to Assist Alzheimer's Caregivers*, published in 1997 and available through its chapters, is helpful. The Patient Locator Unit has been developed to locate people within a 6- to 10-mile range using a 25-kHz frequency allocation (Melillo & Futrell, 1998).

## REFERENCES

Alessi, C.A. (1991). Managing the behavioral problems of dementia in the home. *Clinics in Geriatric Medicine, 7*, 787–801.

Dickinson, J.I., McLain-Kark, J., & Marshall-Baker, A. (1995). The effects of visual barriers on exiting behavior in a dementia care unit. *Gerontologist, 35*, 127–130.

Hewawasam, L. (1996). Floor patterns limit wandering of people with Alzheimer's. *Nursing Times, 92*(23), 41–44.

Holmberg, S.K. (1997a). Evaluation of a clinical intervention for wanderers on a geriatric nursing unit. *Archives of Psychiatric Nursing, 11,* 21–28.

Holmberg, S.K. (1997b). A walking program for wanderers: Volunteer training and development of an evening walker's group. *Geriatric Nursing, 18*(4), 160–165.

Logsdon, R.G., Teri, L., McCurry, S.M., Gibbons, L.E., Kukull, W.A., & Larson, E.B. (1998). Wandering: A significant problem among community-residing individuals with Alzheimer's disease. *Journal of Gerontology, 53,* P294–P299.

Matteson, M.A., & Linton, A. (1996). Wandering behaviors. *Journal of Gerontological Nursing, 22*(9), 39–46.

Melillo, K.D., & Futrell, M. (1998). Wandering and technology devices. *Gerontological Nursing, 24*(8), 32–34.

Ryan, J.P., McGowan, J., McCaffrey, N., Ryan, T., Zandi, T., & Brannigan, G.G. (1995). Graphomotor perseveration and wandering and Alzheimer's disease. *Journal of Geriatric Psychiatry and Neurology, 8,* 209–212.

Silverstein, N.L., & Flaherty, G. (1996). Deadly mix: Dementia and wandering. *Gerontologist, 36,* 156–157.

Simard, J. (1999). Making a positive difference in the lives of nursing home residents with Alzheimer's disease: The lifestyle approach. *Journal of Alzheimer Disease and Associated Disorders, 13* (Special Supplement 1), S67–S72.

Strumpf, N.E., Robinson, J.P., Wagner, J.S., & Evans, L.K. (1998). *Restraint-free care: Individualized approaches for frail elders.* New York: Springer.

Volicer, L., Brandeis, G.H., & Hurley, A.C. (1998). Infections in advanced dementia. In L. Volicer & A. Hurley (Eds.), *Hospice care for patients with advanced progressive dementia* (pp. 29–47). New York: Springer.

Warner, M.L. (1998). *The complete guide to Alzheimer's-proofing your home.* West Lafayette, IN: Purdue University Press.

# Glossary

**Acetylcholine**   A chemical that is a neurotransmitter that is used by nerve cells to communicate with each other

**Acetylcholinesterase Inhibitors**   Chemicals that inhibit acetylcholinesterase (an enzyme that breaks down acetylcholine); they increase the effect of remaining acetylcholine and improve memory and, possibly, other cognitive functions.

**Activities of Daily Living (ADLs)**   Those activities that are needed for self-care and independent living; they include instrumental activities of daily living (IADLs) and physical activities of daily living (PADLs).

**ADL Dependence**   Self-care deficit that is caused by the interaction of cognitive and physical impairments and results in the inability to perform normal, routine, daily PADL and IADL functions

**Agitation**   Observed behaviors that are indicative of an unpleasant state of excitement, which remain after interventions to reduce internal or external stimuli have been carried out by alleviating aversive physical signs, managing resistiveness, and decreasing sources of accumulated stress

**Agnosia**   The inability to recognize familiar objects by sight, touch, taste, smell, or sound

---

The definitions included in this glossary are specific for people with dementia and were developed for use with this book. Other sources may provide generic or specific definitions for other disorders.

217

**Alzheimer's Disease**    A type of dementia in which the symptoms show a gradual but relentless progress; histopathology reveals characteristic senile plaques and neurofibrillary tangles. Alzheimer's disease involves memory loss of sufficient severity to interfere with social or occupational functioning and impairments in abstract thinking, judgment, spatial orientation, and/or language.

**Amnesia**    Memory loss

**Anomia**    A problem with naming; part of aphasia

**Anosognosia**    The state in which the person with dementia is unaware of deficits or underestimates the extent of his or her impairment

**Anxiety**    Vague, uneasy feeling with a nonspecific or unknown source; a feeling of distress that is subjectively experienced as a fear or worry and objectively expressed through autonomic and central nervous system responses.

**Apathy**    The state in which a person appears passive, demonstrates inattention to the external environment, or acts uninterested in what is happening around him or her

**Aphasia**    The inability to communicate and/or understand spoken or written words or both; expressive aphasia is the inability to form words or express oneself clearly orally or in writing; receptive aphasia refers to the decreased ability to understand spoken or written language.

**Apraxia**    The inability to initiate purposeful motor functions or use objects properly, or both, despite no known physical problems. The person may be able to perform an activity spontaneously but not "on command." Apraxia results from a breakdown in the pathway in the brain between where an idea for action occurs or a direction is understood, and where it is carried out.

**Ataxia**    A lack of muscle coordination resulting in impaired gait

**Bright Eyes**    Structured sensory stimulation intervention that sequentially invokes the olfactory, kinesthetic, tactile, visual, auditory, and gustatory senses by the use of sensory cues organized around a central theme to elicit adaptive responses to the cue

**Caregiver Guilt**    An emotion that arises from a caregiver's belief that he or she has "failed the person" in his or her care

**Circumlocution**    The use of nonverbal communication or word substitution to avoid revealing that a name or word has been forgotten

**Comorbidity**    The presence of any other distinct additional clinical entity in addition to dementia (Because most other diseases are also more common among older adults, many people with dementia who are elderly may have other chronic diseases associated with old age.)

**Contracture**    Fibrosis, shortening, or tightening of a muscle that prevents the normal mobility of the related tissue or joint

**Delirium**    A temporary state that is characterized by an acute onset of mental status change (fluctuating course; decreased ability to focus, sustain, and shift attention; and either disorganized thinking or an altered level of consciousness) that resolves if the precipitating causes are removed

**Delusions**    False beliefs that are based on incorrect information about an external reality that are firmly sustained despite what almost everyone believes and despite evidence constituting incontrovertible and obvious proof to the contrary

**Dementia**    Any acquired state of decreased mental ability of long duration (months to years) that impairs daily activities in a previously alert individual

**Dementia Special Care Unit**    A formalized area where people with dementia receive care under special guidelines from specially educated staff in an environment that has been adapted to meet their unique needs

**Dementia with Lewy Bodies**    This disease is characterized by a fluctuating course of cognitive impairment that includes episodic confusion and lucid intervals similar to delirium and 1) visual or auditory hallucinations or both resulting in paranoid delusions, 2) mild extrapyramidal symptoms or adverse extrapyramidal response to standard doses of neuroleptics, or 3) repeated unexplained falls; also called diffuse Lewy body disease.

**Depression**    A mental disorder that is marked by symptoms of long-lasting despondent mood often described as overwhelming sadness or emptiness, increase or decrease in appetite or weight, sleeping too much or too little, feeling either agitated or slowed down, loss of interest in usual activities, loss of energy, feeling worthless and guilty, difficulty thinking and concentrating, and thoughts of death or suicide

**Disorientation**    A person's apparent unawareness of or inability to indicate his or her knowledge of time, place, person, or circumstance

**Disruptive Behaviors**    Actions, words, or vocalizations that are perceived by others to be offensive or bothersome

**Drug Holiday**    Taking time off from administering a drug to assess a person's symptoms without pharmacological management to determine whether the drug is still needed for symptom management.

**Elopement**    Leaving a long-term care facility or home without permission

**Engagement**    Attention to people or things in the external environment, such as involvement in a conversation or participation in other meaningful activities

**Excess Disability**    More physical or mental limitation or impairment than can be explained by the underlying disease process

**Executive Function**    Ability to plan and think in abstract terms; loss of executive function may be tested by asking people with dementia to interpret proverbs.

**Food Refusal**    Active or passive rejection of food by ceasing to feed oneself, if able; or by trying to prevent a caregiver from feeding by not opening one's mouth when being fed or by pushing a hand or utensil away

**Force Feeding**    Feeding a person against his or her wishes by either natural or artificial means

**Frontotemporal Dementia**    Symptoms of altered personality that are similar to changes induced by damage to the frontal lobes by other causes (injury, stroke), which include behavioral disinhibition, loss of social or personal awareness, and disengagement with apathy

**Functional Impairment**    Core symptom of dementia that has great potential influence on several peripheral symptoms. Functional impairment has both cognitive and physical components; it creates increasing inability of people with dementia to cope with either environmental or internal stressors. Physical components may be the result of dementia, comorbidities, or disuse.

**Gastrostomy Tube**    A tube that is surgically inserted into the stomach to provide hydration and nutrition for a prolonged period of time

**Graphomotor Perseveration**    Inability to terminate or shift a behavior once it is initiated

**Habilitation**    A proactive therapeutic milieu that emphasizes the importance of emotions in understanding the needs of people with dementia and a positive caregiving attitude aimed at the maintenance of existing function rather than the restoration of lost abilities

**Hallucinations**    Sensory perceptions that occur without the appropriate stimulation of the corresponding sensory organ

**Hospice Approach**   Care that is aimed at providing maximum comfort instead of striving for maximum survival time in the context of a person's previous wishes and family values

**Hyperactivity**   Excessive or continuous motor activity or movement

**Inability to Initiate Meaningful Activities**   The inability to initiate usual, recreational, or leisure activities because of a lack of opportunity or cognitive and physical functional impairments that interfere with the capacity to communicate, engage in activity, and experience and respond to various types of stimulation

**Insomnia**   Prolonged sleep disturbance that may be related to a circadian rhythm disturbance resulting from brain damage in the area of the suprachiasmatic nucleus

**Instrumental Activities of Daily Living (IADLs)**   Those activities that are needed to support independent living and include shopping, preparing meals, traveling, doing housework, using the telephone, taking medication, and managing money

**Intercurrent Illness**   A secondary or concurrent disease, syndrome, or symptoms that occur or coexist in an individual with a separate, usually unrelated, primary medical condition

**Interdisciplinary**   A model of care delivery that stresses collaboration among the wide array of health care providers who perform an assessment, analyze findings, and use data to develop and coordinate a collective goal and plan of care that transcends the view of any single discipline

**Interdisciplinary Team**   A group of health care and social services providers who work together in a collaborative fashion to provide comprehensive, person-focused care for an individual with a complex illness

**Lifestyle Approach**   Framework to help people with dementia adjust to changes in their lives; consists of assessment, implementation, programming, documentation, and evaluation components to provide leisure time that is filled with familiar and meaningful activities

**Merry Walker**   An enclosed metal walker on four wheels with a built-in seat that enhances safety by limiting falls, compensates for decreased endurance by allowing the person to sit down if fatigued, and allows the person to continue mobility in an upright position with modified independence

**Myoclonus**   Sudden repeated retractions of the same muscle

**Neologisms**   Made-up words (e.g., "moombas")

**Pacing**    Repetitively walking back and forth as if following a rhythm or pattern, often with speed and a sense of urgency. Pacing provides exercise; it is merely problematic and should only be limited when it causes fatigue or foot problems or poses a risk of malnutrition because it interferes with sitting down to eat or requires more calories than provided by the person's daily intake.

**Paraphrasia**    Speech that is seemingly incoherent, unintelligible, or incomprehensible but may be meaningful when interpreted by another

**Paratonia**    An involuntary rigidity response, which causes a flexed posture, loss of balance, and falls

**Perseveration**    Repetition of an action without an appropriate stimulus. The person has difficulty terminating a behavior once initiated or experiences an inability to shift to another behavior.

**Physical Activities of Daily Living (PADLs)**    Functional skills, including bathing, dressing, grooming, toileting, walking (mobility), and eating

**Pick's Disease**    Pathological subtype of a frontotemporal dementia; characterized by Pick bodies inside nerve cells and ballooned nerve cells

**Reframing**    Communicating an idea another way by using familiar, comforting, and nonthreatening words or phrases

**Reminiscence**    Process of recalling pleasurable memories; conceptually close to simulated presence therapy. Reminiscence is implemented by storytelling, looking at favorite photo albums, conversation, listening to music, or watching a video.

**Resistiveness to Care (RTC)**    Behaviors used by people with dementia to withstand or oppose the efforts of a caregiver

**Respite**    Any formal support service or treatment intervention aimed at providing temporary physical and emotional relief to the caregiver of a person with dementia

**Sensory Deprivation**    Lack of appropriate levels of stimulation necessary for maintaining normal contact with the environment; often manifested by blunting of affect, reduced spontaneity, apathy, or cognitive impairment

**Sensory Overload**    More stimulation than an individual is able to effectively cope with; often manifested by anxiety, restlessness, agitation, or, in some cases, catastrophic behavioral reactions

**Simulated Presence Therapy**   Also known as SimPres. In simulated presence therapy (SPT), a person's best-loved experiences are selected from his or her long-term memories and are audiotaped by a family member or staff member in the context of a normal, spontaneous conversation that is then played using a headset with an autoreverse tape player, allowing time for the person's responses.

**Snoezelen**   Therapeutic multisensory environmental experience that provides a comfortable, lazy feeling; loosely translated from two Dutch words for "sniff" and "doze." A portable component consists of a combination of music and colored light projected through oil onto a screen. Aromatherapy also is sometimes used in Snoezelen.

**Spatial Disorientation**   Misperceiving immediate surroundings, inability to distinguish a two-dimensional from a three-dimensional object, not being aware of one's setting, or not knowing where one is in relation to the environment

**Sundown Syndrome**   A syndrome that is characterized by the appearance or exacerbation of behavioral symptoms of restlessness, excitement, increased confusion, hallucinations, and/or agitation seen in the late afternoon or early evening

**Supportive Care**   Care that is delivered for the purpose of preserving remaining function and promoting comfort in an individual for whom there is no reasonable hope for complete recovery

**Target Body Weight**   Number of pounds (or kilograms) that the interdisciplinary team has determined is appropriate for a person to weigh based on pertinent assessment factors such as usual body weight, laboratory values, estimated height and body frame, eating behaviors, presence of intercurrent illness, and activity status

**Time-Out**   Termination of attempts of a caregiver to provide care when it is not successful. The caregiver stops, leaves, and then returns and starts fresh with a new approach.

**Validation Therapy**   Framework for caregiver–care recipient interaction that reaffirms the dignity of the person with dementia and the humanity of the health care professional by using empathetic understanding as a communication tool

**Vascular Dementia**   Dementia symptoms caused by multiple small or large brain infarcts, or both, or a small, strategically placed stroke; characterized by an abrupt onset, focal neurological findings, and low-density areas, presence of multiple strokes, or both on computerized tomography scans or magnetic resonance imaging

# Index

Page numbers followed by *f* indicate figures;
those followed by *t* indicate tables.

ABCs of behavior analysis, 142–143
Acetylcholine, 23, 24, 52, 69, 217
Acetylcholinesterase inhibitors, 5,
    23–24, 69, 217
Activities of daily living (ADLs), 6,
    79–89, 217
  assessment of functional status,
    80–84
  dependence in, 2, 2*f*, 29, 84–89, 217
  effects of spatial disorientation on,
    130–131, 131*f*
  instrumental, 6, 79, 81–82, 221
  interventions to promote functional
    performance, 80, 86–89, 87*t*
  physical, 6, 79, 82–84, 222
  resistiveness during, 145–146
Activity-planning strategies, 95–104
  documenting responses to interven-
    tions, 104–105
  for early to moderate stages of
    dementia, 98–101
    cognitive activities, 98
    diversional activities, 99–100
    exercise, 101
    functional household activities, 99

    reminiscence, 100
    Video Respite®, 100
  guidelines for choosing activities,
    96–98, 97*t*
  for moderate to late stages of demen-
    tia, 101–104
    animal-assisted therapy, 103
    Bright Eyes, 102, 103*t*
    Merry Walker, 103–104
    music, 101–102
    reminiscence, 103
    simulated presence therapy, 101
    Snoezelen, 104
Adapin, *see* Doxepin
Adjustment disorder with depressed
    mood, 6, 49
ADLs, *see* Activities of daily living
Adult day services, 189–190, 194, 195
Age, effects of on sleep, 174–176,
    175*f*
  medical conditions of older adults,
    176
  sleep fragmentation, 174
  sleep-related motor disorders,
    175–176

Age—*continued*
  sleep-related respiratory disorders,
    174–175
Agitation, 2, 2*f*, 8, 187, 190–196, 217
  apathy and, 190
  assessment for causes of, 190
  depression and, 195–196
  physical causes of, 191–195
  rationale for therapeutics for,
    192*t*–194*t*, 196–202
    caregivers, 199–200
    medications, 197–199
    model of psychological well-being,
      196–197, 197*f*
    simulated presence therapy,
      200–201
    sundown syndrome, 201–202
Agnosia, 5, 37–38, 162, 217
  visual, 128, 129
Alprazolam, 121*t*
Aluminum, exposure to, 21–22
Alzheimer's Association Safe Return
  Program, 214
Alzheimer's disease, 5, 218
  diagnosis of, 16–18
  environmental factors and, 3, 20–22
    early life experiences, 21
    estrogen deficiency, 21
    head trauma, 20–21
    low level of education, 21
    toxins, 21–22
  genetic factors and, 19–20
  incidence of, 1
  neurochemistry of, 69
  neuropathology of, 16–17
  personality changes in, 13
  prevention and treatment of, 22–24
    acetylcholinesterase inhibitors,
      23–24
    free radical scavengers, 23
    hormone replacement therapy, 22
  stages of, 3, 4*f*
  vascular dementia and, 15, 18
Ambien, *see* Zolpidem
Amitriptyline, 53, 53*t*
Amnesia, 218; *see also* Memory impairment

β-Amyloid protein, 16, 20–21, 23, 24
Analgesics, 150
"Anger attacks," 61
Animal-assisted therapy, 6, 103
Anomia, 37, 218
Anorexia, 163, 164*t*, 167
Anosognosia, 15, 218
Anticholinergic drugs, 12
Antidepressants, 6, 52–54, 53*t*, 61–62
  for depression with agitation, 196,
    197, 202
  for insomnia, 184
  monoamine oxidase inhibitors, 53
  other, 54
  selective serotonin reuptake
    inhibitors, 54
  tricyclics, 52–53
Antihypertensive agents, 12
Anti-inflammatory drugs, 20
Anxiety, 2, 2*f*, 6–7, 109–122, 218
  assessment of, 114–115, 115*t*
  clinical indicators of, 114–115, 115*t*
  dementia and, 110–111
  effects of on sleep, 178–179
  etiologies and outcomes of, 111–114,
    112*f*
    anxiety as stress response,
      113–114
    anxiety as symptom of illness,
      112–113, 113*t*
    primary anxiety disorders, 111
  in older adults, 109–110
  therapeutic goals and interventions
    for, 116–122
    behavioral, 118–119
    environmental, 116–118, 117*t*
    pharmacological, 119–122, 120*t*,
      121*t*
Anxiolytic medications, 7, 119–122,
  120*t*, 122*t*
Apathy, 2*f*, 8, 187–190, 200, 218
  agitation and, 190
  depression and, 188–189
  engagement and, 189–190
  *see also* Inability to initiate meaning-
    ful activities
Aphasia, 5, 32–35, 162, 218

Apnea, sleep, 174–175
Apolipoprotein E, 17, 20, 58
Appetite loss, 163, 164t
Appetite stimulants, 167
Apraxia, 5, 36–37, 218
Aricept, *see* Donepezil
Assaultive behavior, 191, 195
Assessment
  of anxiety, 114–115, 115t
  for causes of agitation, 190–191
  of cognitive function, 30–31
  for dementia, 14–19
  of functional status, 80–84
  of people at risk for resistiveness,
    142–146
Ataxia, 218
Ativan, *see* Lorazepam
Aventyl, *see* Nortriptyline

BANS-S, *see* Bedford Alzheimer Nurs-
    ing Severity Scale
Bathing, 88
  to improve sleep, 183
  resistiveness to, 145–146
  techniques for, 147, 147f, 148f
Bedford Alzheimer Nursing Severity
    Scale (BANS-S), 31
Behavior analysis, 142–143
Behavioral interventions
  for anxiety, 118–119
  for delusions and hallucinations, 71
  for elopement, 211–212
  for inability to initiate meaningful
    activities, 95–104
  for insomnia, 180–181, 181t
  for mood disorders, 55
  for resistiveness to care, 147–150
Benign senile forgetfulness, 14–15
Benzodiazepines
  for anxiety, 120, 121t
  for delusions and hallucinations, 73t,
    75
  for insomnia, 184
  paradoxical reaction to, 184
Benztropine, 12
Bipolar disorders, 6, 51–52

dementia and, 60–61
epidemiology of, 48
mood stabilizers for, 56–58, 57t
types of, 51
Body weight, target, 223
Brain imaging, 14
Brief dynamic psychotherapy, 55–56
Bright Eyes, 6, 102, 103t, 218
Buspar, *see* Buspirone
Buspirone, 120, 121t

Capgras syndrome, 67
Carbamazepine, 57, 57t
Care plan, 166
Caregiving, 3, 199–200
  art and science of, 4
  caregiver guilt, 218
  resistiveness to care and, 144–145
  support for family caregivers,
    202–203
Case studies, 5
Cerebrospinal fluid examination, 16–17
Chloralhydrate, 184
Choking, 162
Cholinesterase inhibitors, 5, 23–24, 69,
    217
Chronobiological strategies for insom-
    nia, 181–183
  increasing daytime physical activity,
    183
  light therapy, 182–183
  passive heating, 183
Cimetidine, 12
Circadian rhythm, 172–173
  abnormalities in dementia, 177, 182
  chronobiological strategies for
    insomnia, 181–183
  genetic factors and, 173
  phase advance or delay, 173
  sundowning and, 202
Circumlocution, 33, 34, 218
Clonazepam, 121t
Clozapine, 74
Clozaril, *see* Clozapine
Cognex, *see* Tacrine
Cognitive activities, 98

Cognitive impairment, 30–39
    agnosia, 37–38
    aphasia, 32–35
    apraxia, 36–37
    assessment for, 30–31
    executive functions, 32
    intervention strategies for, 38–39
        mild to moderate stages, 39
        moderate to severe stages, 39
    short-term memory loss, 31–32
Cognitive mapping, 127–128
Cognitive Performance Test (CPT),
    81–82
Cognitive therapy, 55, 71
Combative behavior, 2f, 191, 195
Communication strategies
    aphasia and, 32–35
    delusions and hallucinations and,
        72
Comorbidity, 5, 41, 219
Continuous positive airway pressure
    (CPAP), 176
Contractures, 219
CPAP, see Continuous positive airway
    pressure
CPT, see Cognitive Performance Test
CSF examination, see Cerebrospinal
    fluid examination
Cue navigation, 128
Cues, pop-up, 129
Cyclothymic disorder, 51


Day services, adult, 189–190, 194, 195
Delirium, 5, 11–12, 66, 219
Delusions and hallucinations, 1, 2, 2f,
    6, 12, 65–75
    conditions associated with, 66–67
    definitions of, 66, 219, 220
    drug-induced, 66–67
    effects of on sleep, 184–185
    epidemiology of, 67–68
    etiology of, 68–70
    paranoid delusions, 65–67
    prevalence of in Alzheimer's disease,
        66

relationship to other behavioral
        symptoms of dementia, 70
    spatial disorientation and, 130
    treatment of, 71–75
        medications, 73–75, 73t
        nonpharmacological, 71–73
Dementia, 219
    core consequences and secondary
        symptoms of, 1–3, 2f
    delirium and, 11–12
    diagnostic workup for, 14–19
    due to more than one mechanism,
        15, 17f
    effect of on sleep, 177–178
    frontotemporal, 5, 13, 19, 220
    irreversible, 16t
    with Lewy bodies, 5, 219
        diagnosis of, 18
        hallucinations in, 67–68
    mood disorders and, 58–61
    onset of, 15–16
    personality and, 12–14, 24–25
    potentially reversible, 15t
    progressive, 1
    special care unit, 219
    stages of, 3–4, 4f
    symptom management for, 3
    vascular, 5, 15, 18, 224
Depakene, see Valproic acid
Depakote, see Valproic acid
Dependence in activities of daily living,
        2, 2f, 29, 84–89, 217
    factors affecting, 84–86
        contextual factors, 85
        core symptoms, 84–85
        risk factors for decline, 85–86
    interventions to promote functional
        performance, 80, 86–89, 87t
    see also Activities of daily living
Depression, 2, 5–6, 47–62, 219
    agitation and, 195–196
    apathy and, 188–189
    consequences in advanced dementia,
        61–62
    effects of on sleep, 178–179, 184
    epidemiology of, 47–48

relationship between dementia and, 58–60
  degenerative dementia without depression, 59
  depression in degenerative dementia, 59–60
  depressive dementia, 59
  independent co-occurrence, 60
  major depression without depressive dementia, 59
suicide and, 48
symptoms of, 48
treatment of, 52–58
  antidepressants, 52–54, 53t, 61–62
  electroconvulsive therapy, 52, 56
  mood stabilizers, 52, 56–58, 57t
  psychotherapy, 52, 54–56
types of, 48–51, 50t
  adjustment disorder with depressed mood, 49
  atypical depression, 49
  depressive disorder not otherwise specified, 49–50
  dysthymic disorder, 49, 50t
  major depressive disorder, 49, 50t
  psychotic depression, 49, 66
  seasonal affective disorder, 49
Depth perception, 128
Desipramine, 58
Desyrel, see Trazodone
Devices to prevent elopement, 213–214
Diagnosis, 14–19
  of Alzheimer's disease, 16–18
  of dementia with Lewy bodies, 18
  of frontotemporal dementia, 19
  of vascular dementia, 18
Diagnostic and Statistical Manual of Mental Disorders, 12, 51, 111
Diazepam, 75
Diffuse Lewy body disease, see Dementia, with Lewy bodies
Digoxin, 12
Diphenhydramine, 12
Disability, excess, 220
Discomfort Scale, 150
Disorientation, 219

spatial, 2, 2f, 7, 125–137, 223
Disruptive behaviors, 2f, 219; see also individual types
Distraction, 149
Diversional activities, 99–100
Diversional activity deficit, 94
Donepezil, 23–24, 176, 178
Dopamine, 69, 176
Doxepin, 53, 53t, 184
Dressing, 88
Driving, 133
Drug holiday, 120, 220
Dysphoria, 188; see also Depression
Dysthymic disorder, 6, 49, 50t

Early life experiences, 21
Eating, 89, 155–169
  environmental factors and, 159–160, 165t
  guidelines for promotion of, 155–161
  managing food refusal through stages of dementia, 161–162
  nourishment plan, 158–159
  preventing/breaking cycle of behaviors used to refuse food, 163–167, 164t–166t
  preventing consequences of food refusal in terminal stage of dementia, 168–169
  problems caused by dementia, 157–158
  safety and, 159, 159t
  shaping process of, 160–161
  utensils for, 159
Eating Behavior Scale, 89
ECT, see Electroconvulsive therapy
Educational level, 21
EEG, see Electroencephalography
Effexor, see Venlafaxine
Elavil, see Amitriptyline
Elderly population, 1
Electroconvulsive therapy (ECT), 6, 52, 56
Electroencephalography (EEG), 14
  sleep, 171, 172t

Electroencephalography (EEG)—
    *continued*
    in dementia, 177
    in depression and anxiety, 178
Elopement, 2*f,* 8, 13, 205–214, 220
    explanatory model for, 209–210, 210
    identification of "lost" people,
        208–209
    pacing, 207–209
    prevalence of, 206
    therapeutic goals and interventions
        for, 210–214
        devices, 213–214
        early intervention program, 214
        environmental modifications,
            212–213
        removing precipitants of elope-
            ment, 211
        strategies based on knowledge of
            individual, 212
        treating underlying causes related
            to dementing illness, 211
        wandering behaviors, 206–207
Endep, *see* Amitriptyline
Engagement, 189–190, 220
Environmental factors, 3, 20–22
    circadian rhythm and, 173
    early life experiences, 21
    eating and, 159–160, 165*t*
    estrogen deficiency, 21
    head trauma, 20–21
    low level of education, 21
    spatial disorientation and, 131*f*
    toxins, 21–22
Environmental interventions, 71
    for anxiety, 116–118
    for elopement, 212–214
    for spatial disorientation, 129–130,
        132–137
Eskalith, *see* Lithium
Estrogen deficiency, 21
Excess disability, 220
Executive functions, 32, 220
Exercise, 6, 42–43, 101
    sleep and, 183

Falling, 43
Fear, *see* Anxiety
Feeding tube, 168–169, 220
Fibromyalgia, 176
Fluoxetine, 53*t,* 54
Fluvoxamine, 53*t,* 54
Food refusal, 2*f,* 7, 155–169, 220
    eating problems caused by dementia,
        157–158
    guidelines for prevention of,
        156–161
    management of, 161–162
        in mild dementia, 161
        in moderate dementia, 161–162
        in severe dementia, 162
        in terminal dementia, 162
    preventing/breaking cycle of behav-
        iors used in, 163–167,
        164*t*–166*t*
    preventing consequences of, in ter-
        minal dementia, 168–169
    strategies to decrease risk of,
        160–161
    *see also* Eating
Force feeding, 220
Free radical scavengers, 5, 23
Frontotemporal dementia, 5, 220
    diagnosis of, 19
    personality changes in, 13
Functional household activities, 99
Functional impairment, 1, 2*f,* 5, 29–44,
        220
    cognitive, 30–39
    physical, 40–44
    risk factors for, 85–86
Functional status assessment, 80–84
    dimensions of functional status,
        80–81
    instrumental activities of daily living,
        81–82
    physical activities of daily living,
        82–84

Gabapentin, 57–58, 57*t*
Gastrostomy tube, 168–169, 220

Gegenhalten, 44
Genetic factors
  in dementia, 19–20
  in regulation of circadian rhythm,
    173
Ginkgo biloba extract, 23
Glucocorticoids, 172
Godot syndrome, 110
Graphomotor perseveration, 220
Growth hormone, 172

Habilitation, 220
Haldol, see Haloperidol
Hallucinations, see Delusions and hal-
    lucinations
Haloperidol, 73–74, 73t
Head trauma, 20–21
Hearing impairment, 95
Heterocyclic antidepressants, 54
Hippocampus, 127–128
Hormone replacement therapy, 5, 21,
    22, 24
Hospice, 221
Housekeeping activities, 99
Human Genome Project, 20
Hyperactivity, 221
Hypomania, 48, 51, 56, 60–61

IADLs, see Instrumental activities of
    daily living
Identification bracelet/jewelry, 208–209
Immobility, 5, 40–41
Inability to initiate meaningful activi-
    ties, 2, 2f, 6, 29, 93–105, 221
  behavior management strategies for,
    95–104
    early to moderate stages of demen-
      tia, 98–101
    guidelines for choosing activities,
      96–98, 97t
    moderate to late stages of demen-
      tia, 101–104
  documenting responses to interven-
    tions for, 104–105
  health status and, 95

see also Activity-planning strategies
Insomnia, 2f, 7–8, 179–185, 221
  behavioral strategies for, 180–181
    sleep-restriction therapy, 181
    stimulus control, 180–181, 181t
  lifestyle changes for, 179–180
  see also Sleep
Instrumental activities of daily living
    (IADLs), 6, 79, 81–82, 221
Intercurrent illness, 221
Interdisciplinary approach, 221
Interdisciplinary team, 166–167, 221
Interference with other residents, 2f,
    205–214; see also Elopement
Interpersonal psychotherapy, 55
Intervention strategies
  for agitation, 192t–194t, 196–202
  for anxiety, 116–122
  for cognitive impairment, 38–39
  for delusions and hallucinations,
    71–75
  for elopement, 210–214
  for inability to initiate meaningful
    activities, 95–104
  for mood disorders, 52–58
  for physical impairment, 41–44
  to promote functional performance,
    86–89, 87t
  for spatial disorientation, 129–130,
    132–137
  see also Prevention
Irritability, 195

Klonopin, see Clonazepam

Labeling clothing, 208
Language barriers, 206
Language comprehension, 34
Levodopa, 69
Lewy bodies, see Dementia, with Lewy
    bodies
Lifestyle approach, 221
Light therapy, 182–183
Limbic system, 68–69
Lithium, 56, 57t

Lithobid, *see* Lithium
Lorazepam, 73*t*, 75, 120–121, 121*t*
Low-salt diet, 157, 158
Loxapine, 73*t*
Loxitane, *see* Loxapine
Luvox, *see* Fluvoxamine

$\alpha_2$-Macroglobulin, 20
Magnetic resonance imaging (MRI), 14, 21
Major depressive disorder, 49, 50*t*; *see also* Depression
Major histocompatibility complex, 20
Mania, 48, 51, 56, 60–61; *see also* Bipolar disorders
MAOIs, *see* Monoamine oxidase inhibitors
MDS, *see* Minimum Data Set
Mealtimes, 158–159; *see also* Eating
Medic Alert Program, 214
Medications, 1, 3–5
    acetylcholinesterase inhibitors, 23–24, 69, 217
    administered on "as needed" basis, 151
    for agitation, 197–199
    analgesics, 150
    antidepressants, 52–54, 53*t*, 61–62
    anxiolytics, 119–122, 120*t*, 121*t*
    benzodiazepines, 73*t*, 75, 120, 121*t*
    delirium induced by, 12, 66–67
    for delusions and hallucinations, 73–75, 73*t*
    free radical scavengers, 23
    hormone replacement therapy, 21, 22, 24
    for insomnia, 183–185
    mood stabilizers, 52, 56–58, 57*t*
    neuroleptics, 69, 73–75, 73*t*, 184–185
    for resistiveness to care, 150–152
Melatonin, 172–174
Mellaril, *see* Thioridazine
Memory impairment, 12–15, 65
    benign senile forgetfulness, 14–15
    short-term, 31–32

Merry Walker, 6, 43, 87, 103–104, 221
Metrifonate, 69
Mini-Mental Status Examination (MMSE), 30–31
Minimum Data Set (MDS), 83–84
Mirtazapine, 53*t*, 54
MMSE, *see* Mini-Mental Status Examination
Monoamine oxidase inhibitors (MAOIs), 53, 53*t*
Mood disorders, 1, 2*f*, 5–6, 47–62
    consequences of depression in advanced dementia, 61–62
    epidemiology of, 47–48
    relationship with dementia, 58–61
        depression, 58–60
        manic and hypomanic episodes, 60–61
    treatment of, 52–58
        antidepressants, 52–54, 53*t*, 61–62
        electroconvulsive therapy, 52, 56
        mood stabilizers, 52, 56–58, 57*t*
        psychotherapy, 52, 54–56
    types of, 48–52
        bipolar disorder, 51–52
        depressive disorders, 48–51
    *see also* Bipolar disorders; Depression
Mood stabilizers, 6, 52, 56–58, 57*t*
    carbamazepine, 57
    gabapentin, 57–58
    lithium, 56
    valproic acid, 56–57
Motor disorders, sleep-related, 175–176
    in dementia, 177–178
MRI, *see* Magnetic resonance imaging
Music, 6, 7, 101–102, 118–119, 149–150
Mutism, 35
Myoclonus, 221

Nardil, *see* Phenelzine
Nefazodone, 53*t*, 54
Neologisms, 221
Neuritic plaques, 16, 17
Neurofibrillary tangles, 16, 17
Neuroleptics, 69, 73–75, 73*t*, 184–185

Neurontin, *see* Gabapentin
Neuropathology, 16–19
    of Alzheimer's disease, 16–17
    of dementia with Lewy bodies, 18
    of frontotemporal dementia, 19
    physical impairments related to, 40
    spatial disorientation and, 127–129
    of vascular dementia, 18
Neuropsychiatric Inventory, 188
Nightmares, 178
Nortriptyline, 53, 53*t*
Nourishment plan, 157–159
Nursing Home Reform Act, *see*
        Omnibus Budget Reconciliation
        Act of 1987

Obesity, sleep-related respiratory disor-
        ders and, 175
Olanzapine, 73*t*, 74–75, 185
Omnibus Budget Reconciliation Act of
        1987, 80, 120
Oppositional behaviors, *see* Resistive-
        ness to care
Osteoarthritis, 176
Oxazepam, 73*t*, 75, 121*t*

Pacing, 8, 207–209, 222
PADLs, *see* Physical activities of daily
        living
Pain management, 150
Pamelor, *see* Nortriptyline
Paraphrasia, 34, 222
Paratonia, 40, 44, 222
Parkinson's disease, 18, 66, 69, 176,
        177
Parnate, *see* Tranylcypromine
Paroxetine, 53*t*, 54
Passive heating, for insomnia, 183
Patient Locator Unit, 214
Paxil, *see* Paroxetine
Periodic leg movements in sleep,
        175–176
Perseveration, 222
    graphomotor, 220
Personality, 1, 12–14, 24–25

PES-AD, *see* Pleasant Events Schedule-
        Alzheimer's Disease
PET, *see* Positron emission tomography
Pet therapy, *see* Animal-assisted therapy
Phase advance or delay, 173
Phenelzine, 53*t*
Philosophy of care, 3
Physical activities of daily living
        (PADLs), 6, 79, 82–84, 222
Physical impairment, 40–44
    comorbidity and, 41
    immobility, 40–41
    intervention strategies for, 41–44
        mild to moderate stages, 42–43
        moderate to severe stages, 43
        terminal stage, 43–44
    related to type of dementia, 40
Pick's disease, 19, 222
Pleasant Events Schedule-Alzheimer's
        Disease (PES-AD), 96
PLST model, *see* Progressively lowered
        stress threshold model
Pop-up cues, 129
Positron emission tomography (PET),
        127
Posterior cingulate gyrus, 127
Prevention
    of agitated behaviors, 192*t*–193*t*
    of food refusal, 156–161, 163–167,
        164*t*–166*t*
    of resistiveness to care, 146–147,
        147*f*, 148*f*
    *see also* Intervention strategies
Progressively lowered stress threshold
        (PLST) model, 114, 116, 117*t*
Prolactin, 172
Prozac, *see* Fluoxetine
Psychological well-being, model of,
        196–197, 197*f*
Psychotherapy for mood disorders, 52,
        54–56
    behavior therapy, 55
    brief dynamic psychotherapy, 55–56
    cognitive therapy, 55
    interpersonal psychotherapy, 55
Psychotic depression, 49, 66

Quetiapine, 73t, 74, 75

RADL, see Refined ADL Assessment
    Scale
Range-of-motion exercises, 43
Rapid eye movement (REM) sleep,
    171–172, 172t
RAPS, see Resident Assessment Proto-
    cols
Recreational activities, 99–100
Refined ADL Assessment Scale (RADL),
    83–84
Reframing, 222
Rehabilitation, 42–43
REM sleep, see Rapid eye movement
    sleep
Remeron, see Mirtazapine
Reminiscence, 6, 7, 100, 103, 119, 222
Repetitive vocalization, 2f, 195
Resident Assessment Protocols (RAPS),
    83
Resistiveness to care (RTC), 2, 2f, 7,
    139–152, 222
  assessment of people at risk for,
      142–146
    ABCs of behavior analysis,
        142–143
    caregiver variables, 144–145
    context of care, 145–146
    variables in people with dementia,
        143–144
  consequences of, 140, 141f
  properties of resistive behaviors,
      140–142, 141f
  symptom management for, 146–152
    behavioral interventions, 147–150
    medications, 150–152
    preventive strategies, 146–147,
        147f, 148f
RESPECT model, 72
Respiratory disorders, sleep-related,
    174–175
  in dementia, 177–178
Respite service, 222
  Video Respite®, 6, 100
Restless leg syndrome, 176

Restlessness, 194, 195; see also Agita-
    tion
Revised Memory and Behavior Problem
    Checklist, 110
Rheumatoid arthritis, 20
Risperdal, see Risperidone
Risperidone, 73t, 74, 122, 184, 185
RTC, see Resistiveness to care

Schizophrenia, 66
SCN, see Suprachiasmatic nucleus
Seasonal affective disorder, 49
  light therapy for, 182
Selective serotonin reuptake inhibitors
    (SSRIs), 53t, 54
Selegiline, 23
Senile plaques, 16, 17
Sensory deprivation, 222
Sensory impairments, 95
Sensory overload, 222
Serax, see Oxazepam
Seroquel, see Quetiapine
Serotonin, 54
Sertraline, 53t, 54, 58, 178, 196, 202
Serzone, see Nefazodone
Simulated presence therapy (SPT), 6,
    101, 200–201, 223
Sinequan, see Doxepin
Sleep, 171–185
  age, effects of on, 174–176, 175f
    medical conditions of older adults,
        176
    sleep fragmentation, 174
    sleep-related motor disorders,
        175–176
    sleep-related respiratory disorders,
        174–175
  dementia, effects of on, 177–178
    sleep-related disorders, 177–178
    stages of sleep, 177
  depression and anxiety effects on,
      178–179
  regulation of, 172–173
  sleep debt, 173
  stages of, 171–172, 172t
  treatment of insomnia, 179–185

behavioral strategies, 180–181, 181t

chronobiological strategies, 181–183

lifestyle changes, 179–180

medications, 183–185

*see also* Insomnia

Sleep restriction therapy, 181

Smoking, 22

Snoezelen, 6, 7, 104, 119, 223

Snoring, 175

Spatial disorientation, 2, 2f, 7, 125–137, 223

basis for interventions for, 129–130

environmental landmarks, 130

pop-up cues, 129

gaining emotional understanding of, 126–127

management of, 132–137

in mild dementia, 132–133

in moderate dementia, 133–134

in severe dementia, 135–137

model of, 130–131, 131f

pathophysiology of, 127–129

wandering and, 212

SPID, *see* Strategies to Promote Independence in Dressing

SPT, *see* Simulated presence therapy

SSRIs, *see* Selective serotonin reuptake inhibitors

Stages of dementia, 3–4, 4f

Stages of sleep, 171–172, 172t

dementia effects on, 177

Stimulus control strategies, for insomnia, 180–181, 181t

Strategies to Promote Independence in Dressing (SPID), 88

Stress

anxiety and, 113–114

minimizing environmental stressors, 116–118, 117t

Stroke, 18

sleep-related respiratory disorders and, 175

Suicide, 48

Sundown syndrome, 184, 201–202, 223

Support groups for family caregivers, 203

Supportive care, 223

Suprachiasmatic nucleus (SCN), 172–174, 182

Swallowing difficulties, 162, 168

Tacrine, 23–24

Tardive dyskinesia, 73–74

Tau protein, 16, 24

Tegretol, *see* Carbamazepine

Television viewing, 199

Thioridazine, 12, 73t, 74, 184

Thyroid-stimulating hormone, 172

Time out, 223

"Toast test," 82

Toileting/continence, 88–89

Toxins, environmental, 21–22

Tranylcypromine, 53t

Trazodone, 53t, 54, 61, 184

Tricyclic antidepressants, 52–53, 53t

Validation therapy, 223

Valium, *see* Diazepam

Valproic acid, 56–57, 57t

Vascular dementia, 5, 224

Alzheimer's disease and, 15, 18

diagnosis of, 18

Vegetative symptoms, 61

Venlafaxine, 53t, 54

Video Respite®, 6, 100

Violent behavior, 191, 195

Vision impairment, 95

Visual agnosia, 128, 129

Visual inattention, 128

Vitamin E, 23, 24

Wandering behaviors, 206–207; *see also* Elopement

Withdrawn behavior, 94, 188–190; *see also* Apathy

"Wizard of Alz," 126

Xanax, *see* Alprazolam

Zoloft, *see* Sertraline
Zolpidem, 184

Zyprexa, *see* Olanzapine